ANATOMY Coloring BOOK

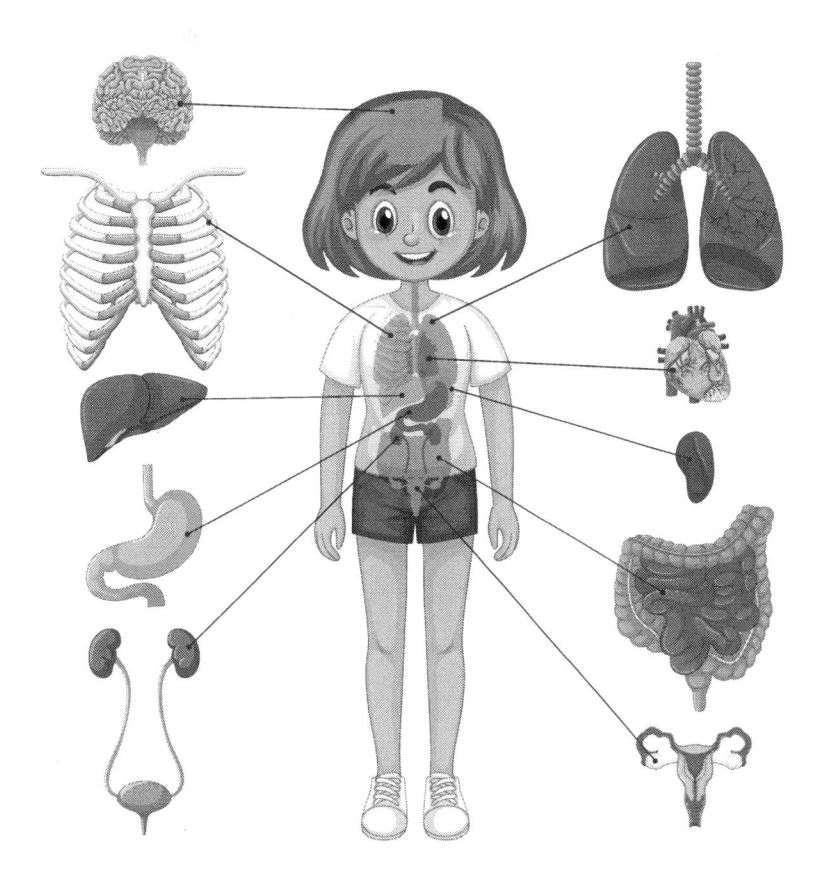

This Book Belongs To

Copyright © 2019

All rights reserved.
No part of this publication
may be reproduced,
distributed, or transmitted
in any form or by any means,
including photocopying, recording,
or other electronic or mechanical
methods, without the prior written
permission of the publisher, except
in the case of brief quotations
embodied in critical reviews and
certain other noncommercial uses
permitted by copyright law.
For permission requests,
write to the publisher.

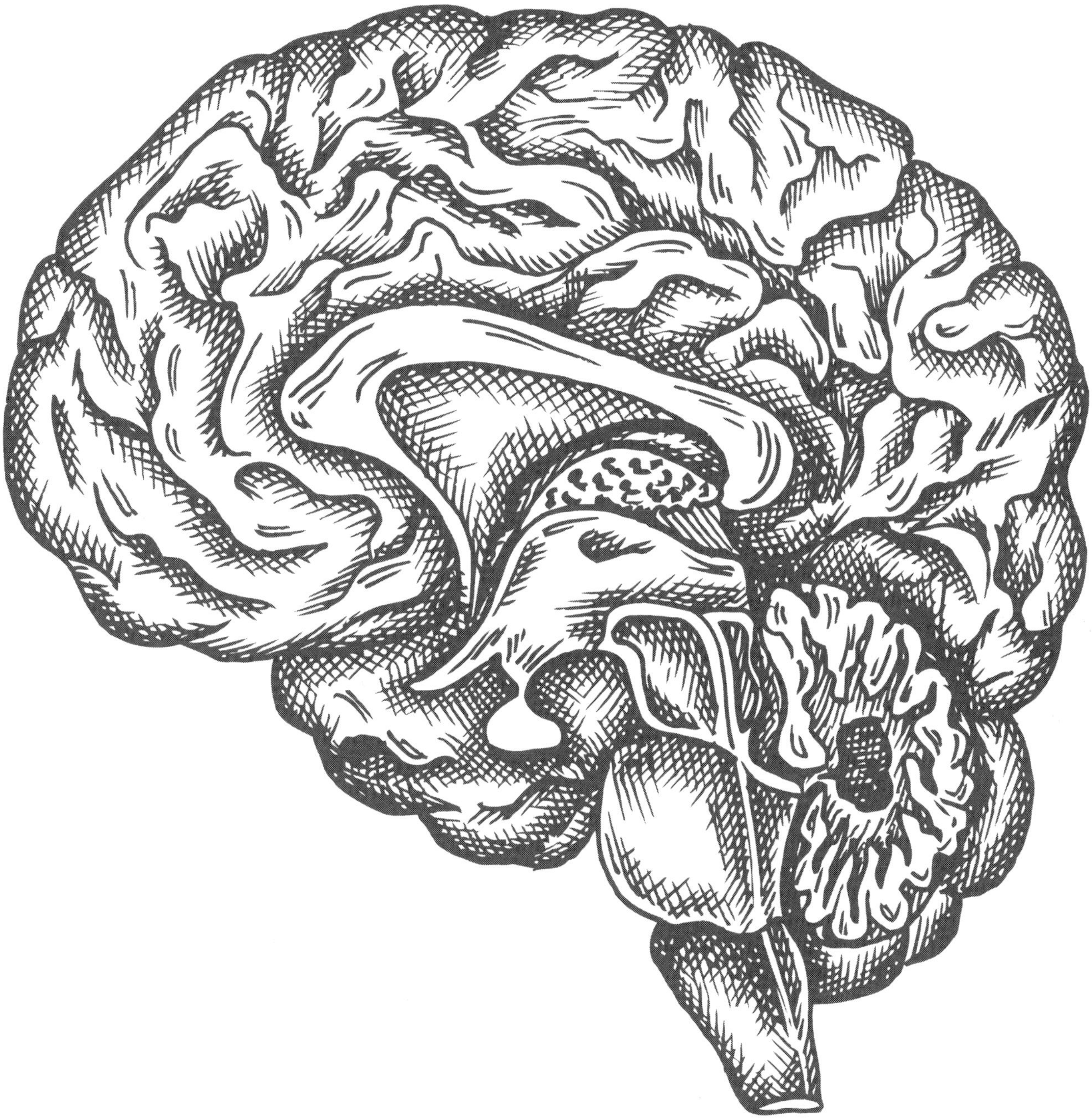

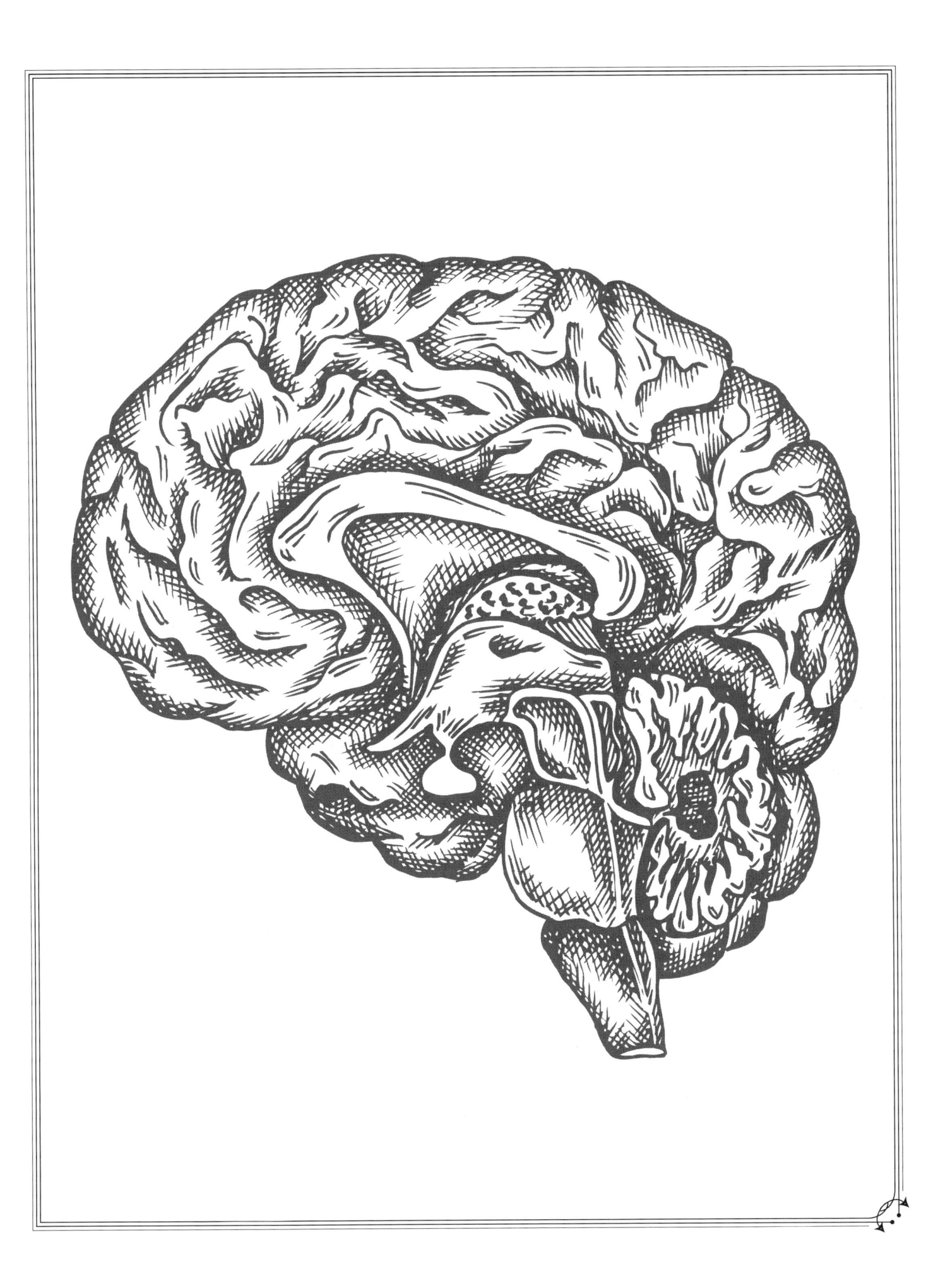

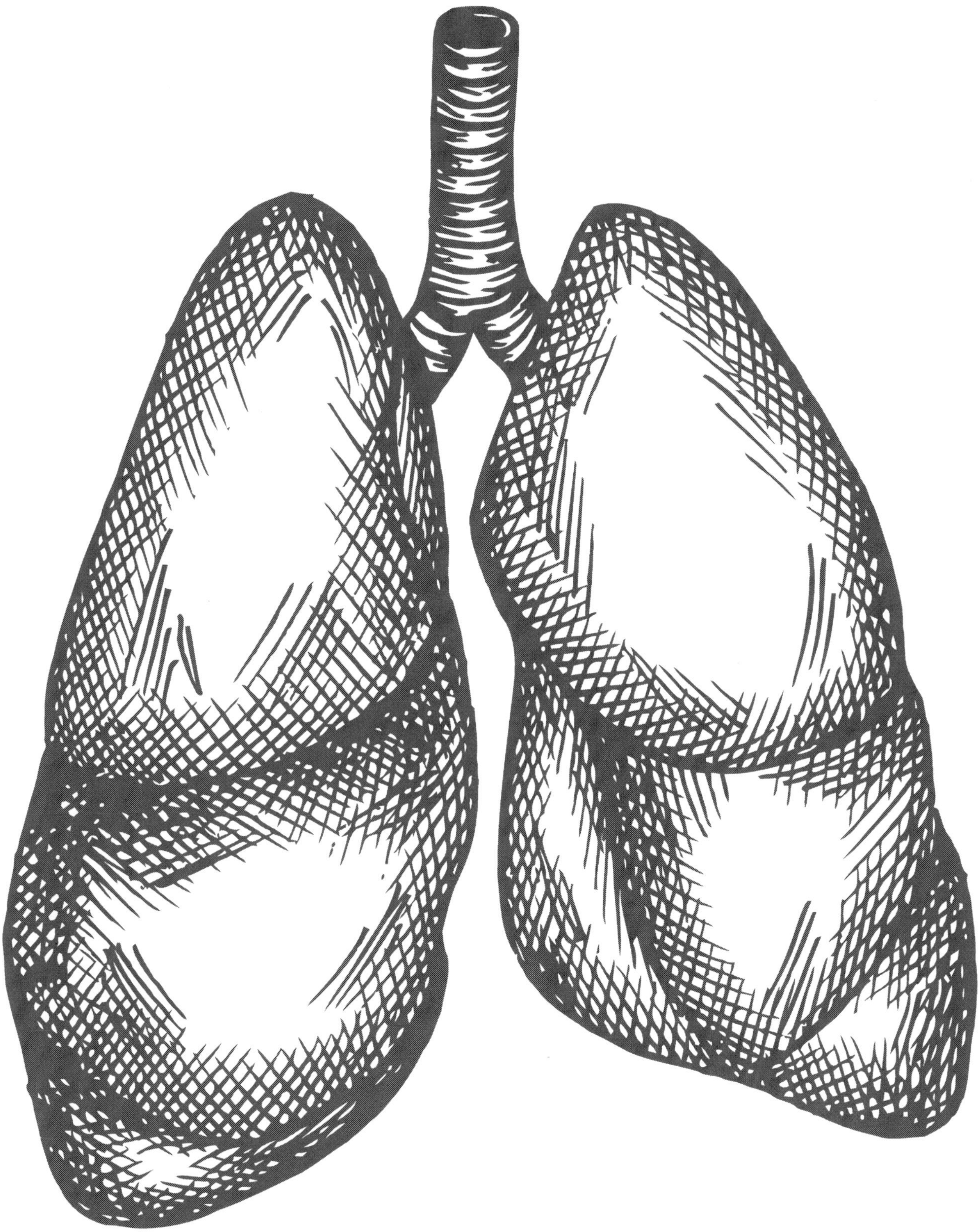

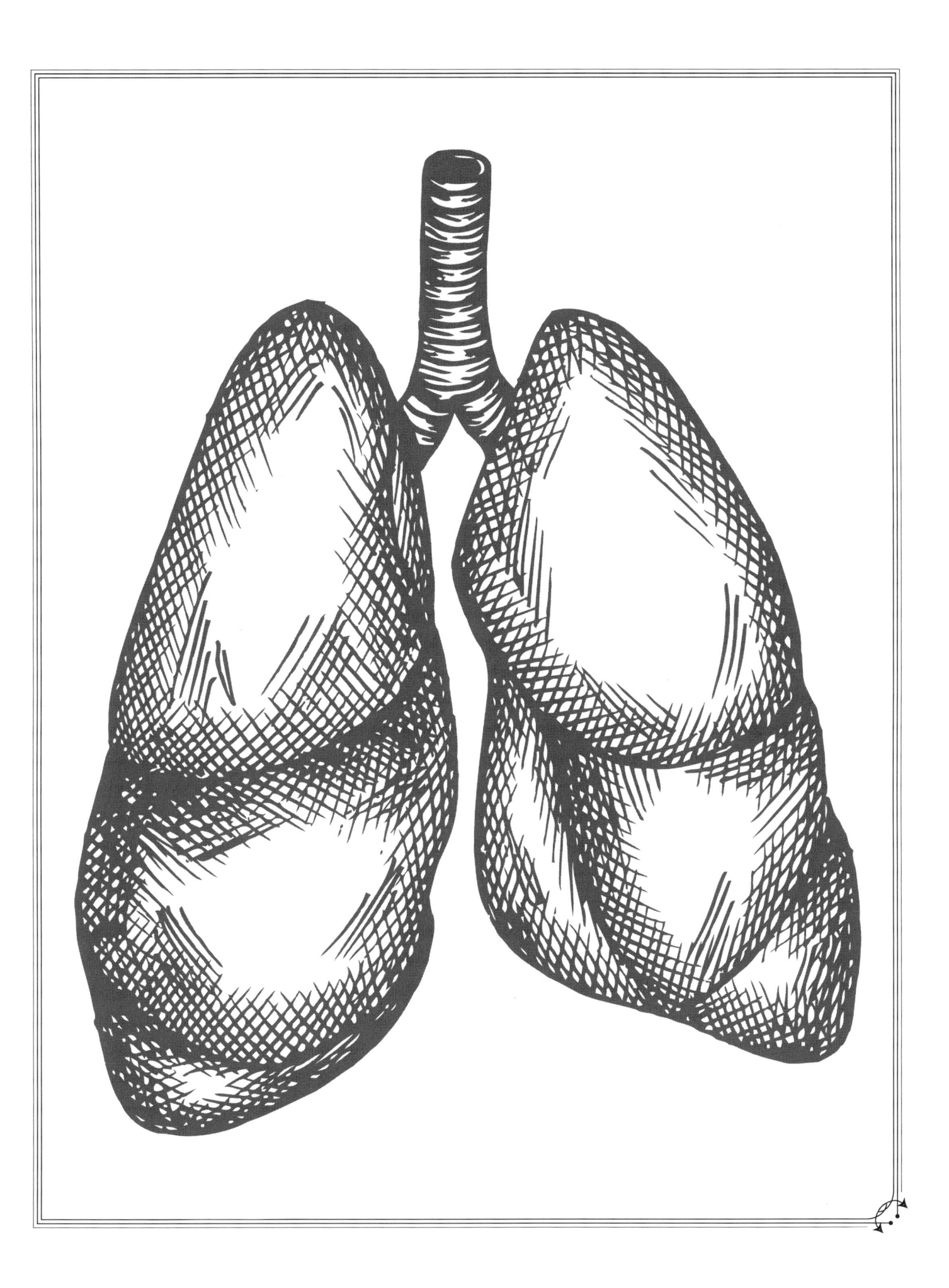

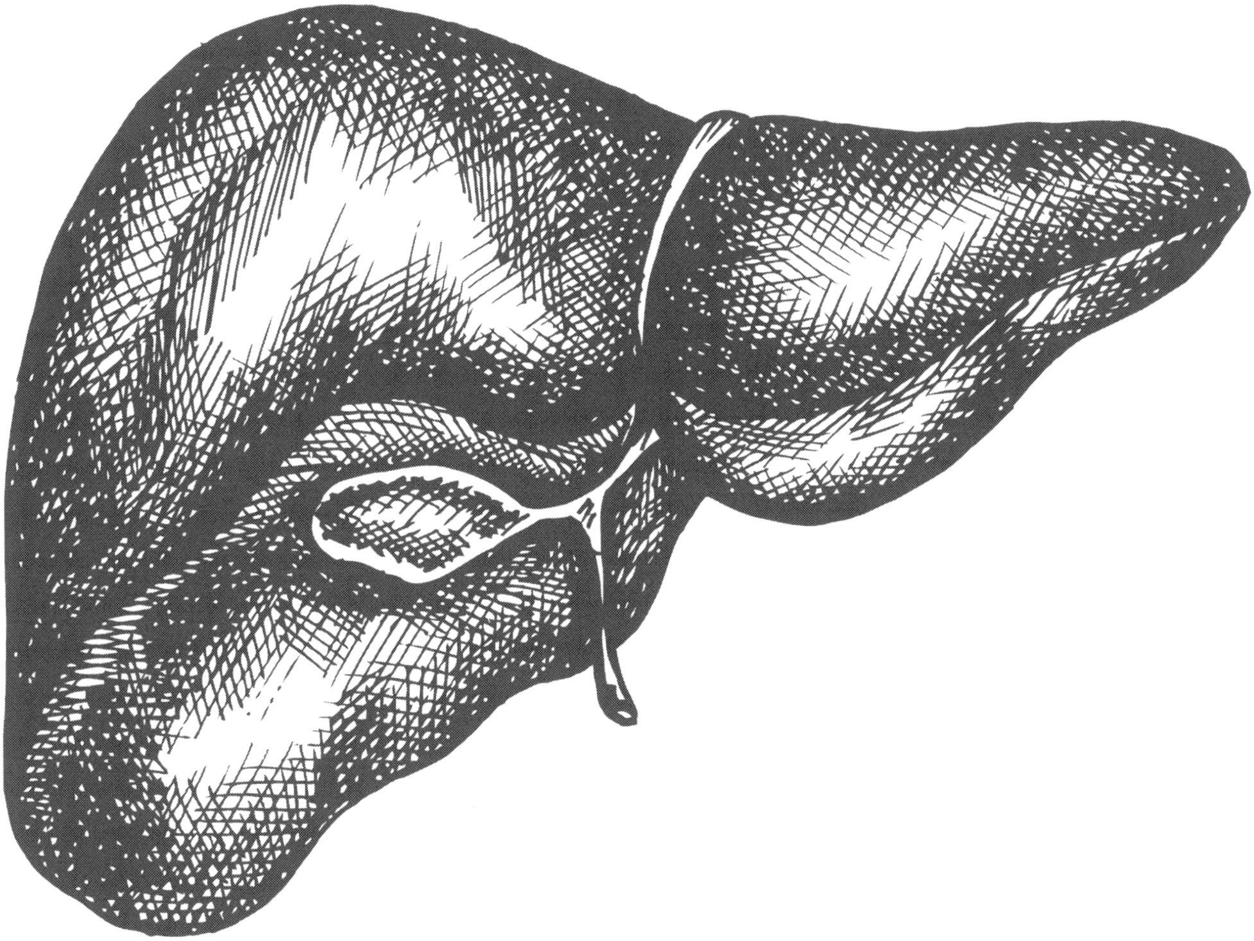

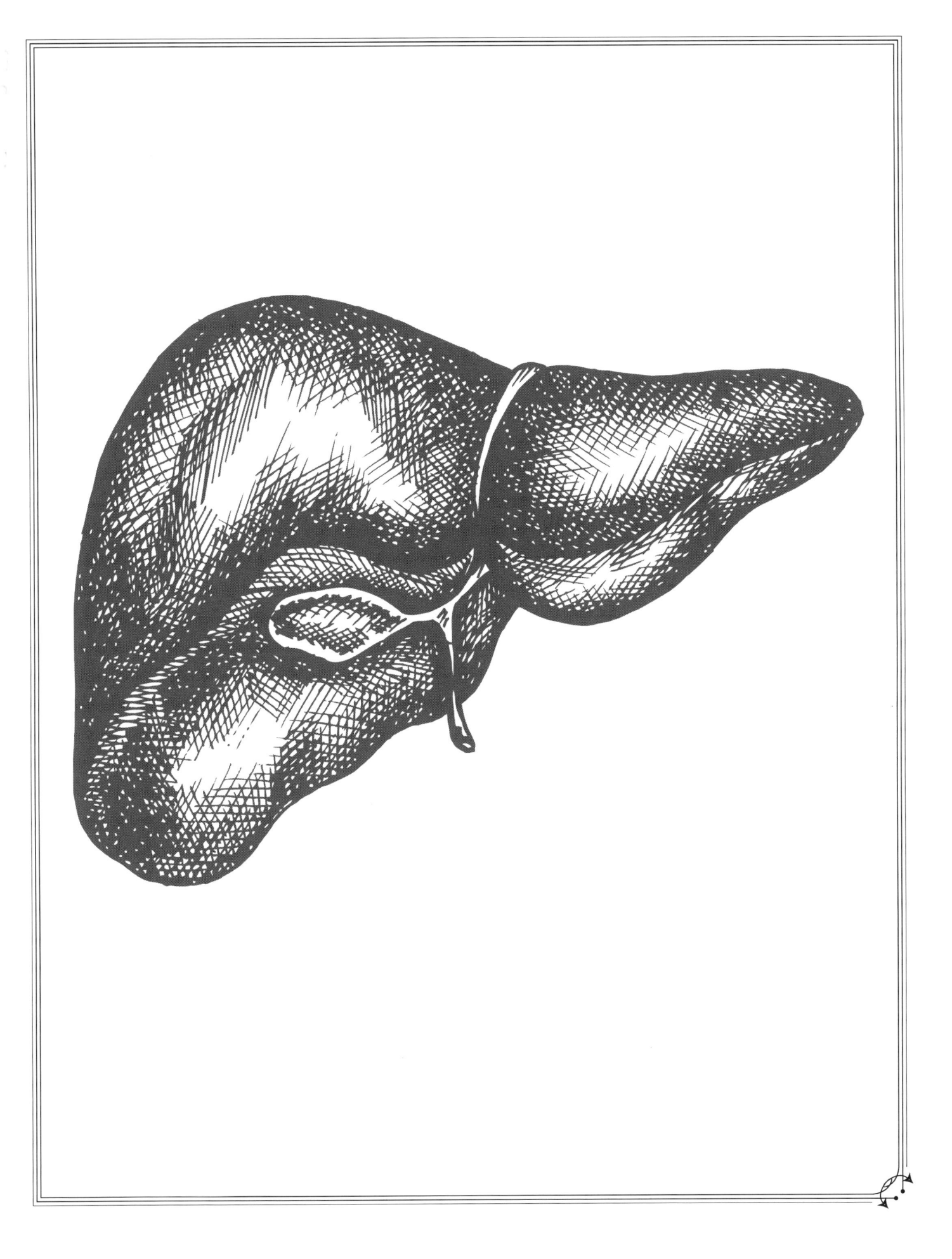

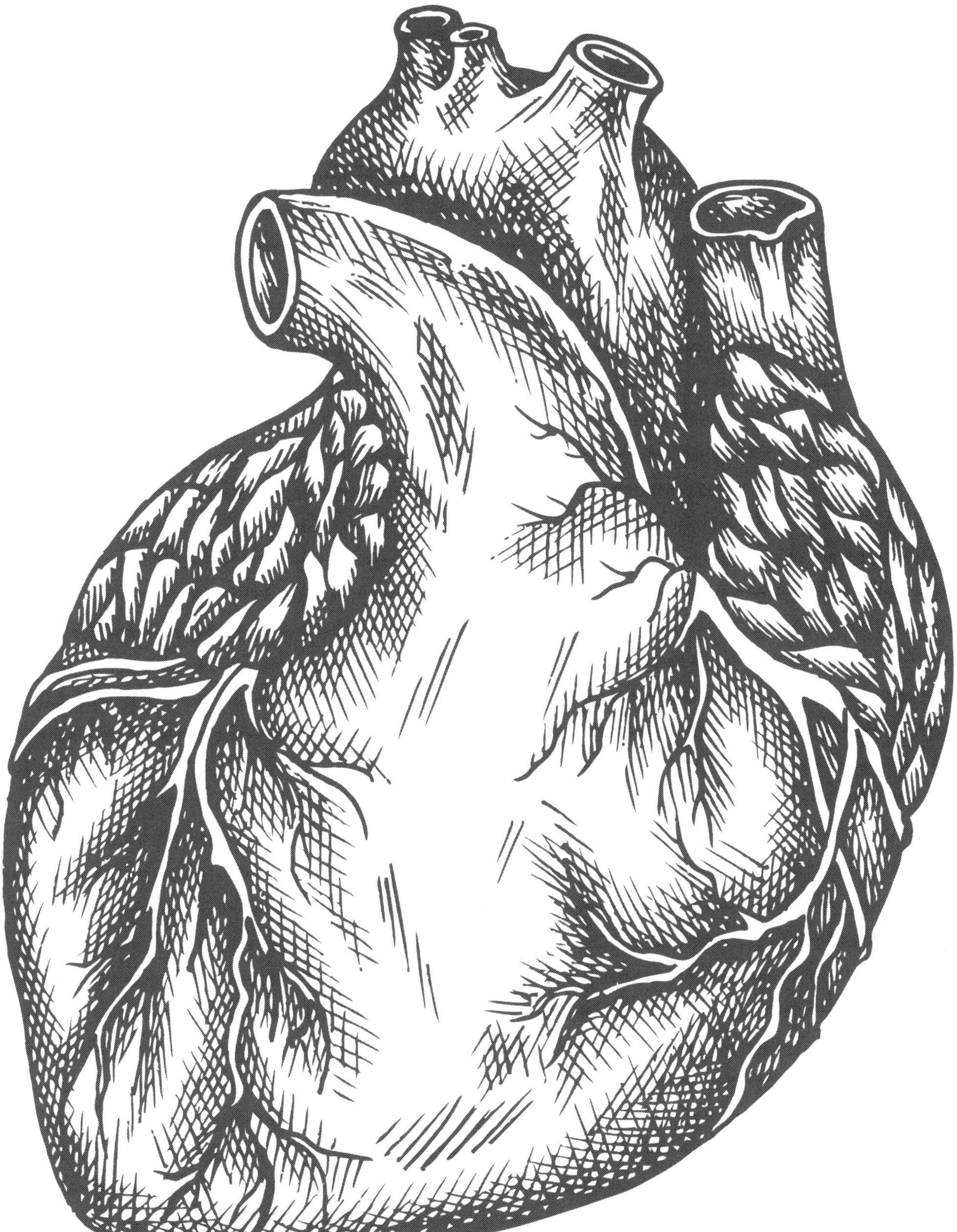

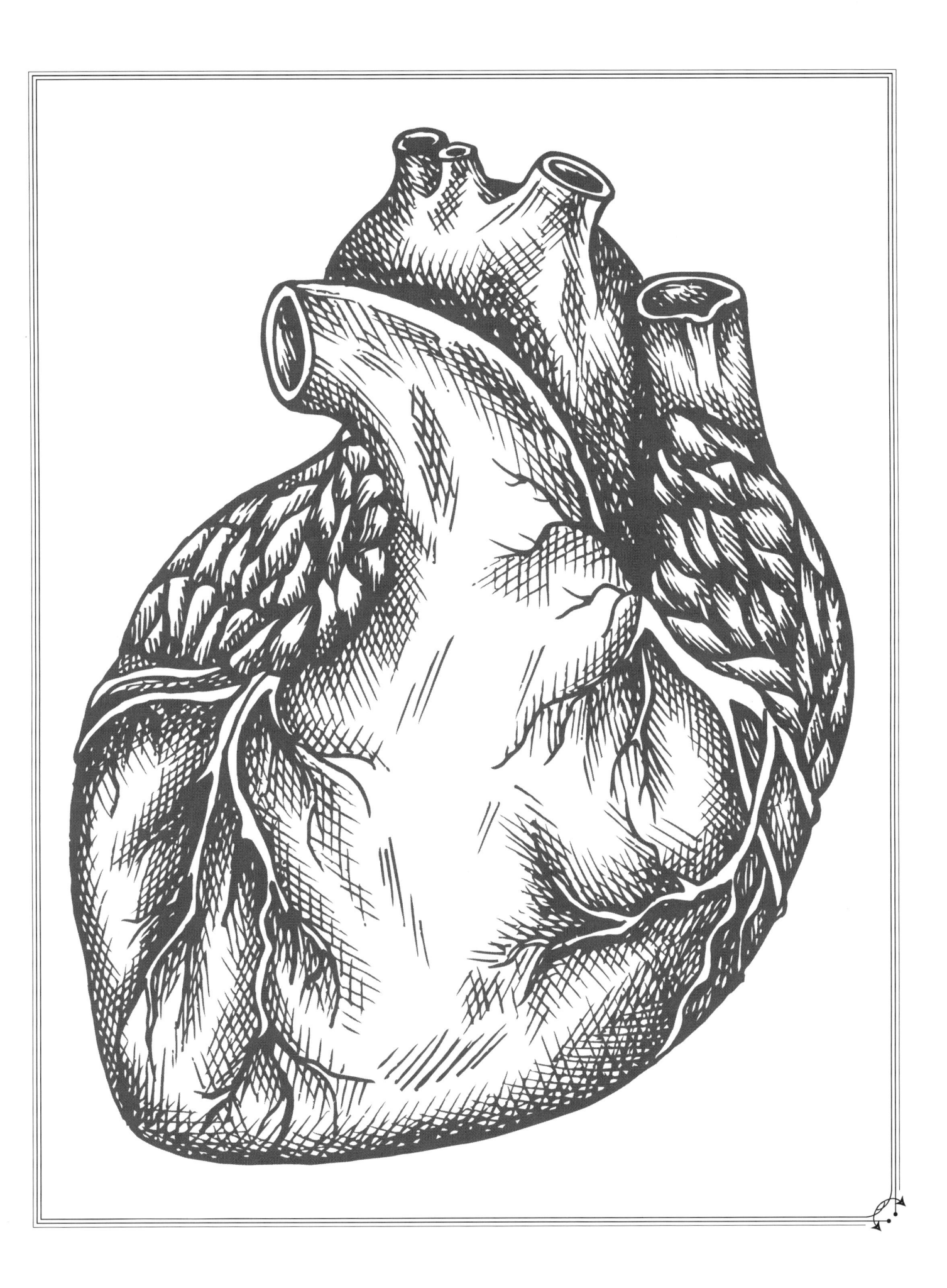

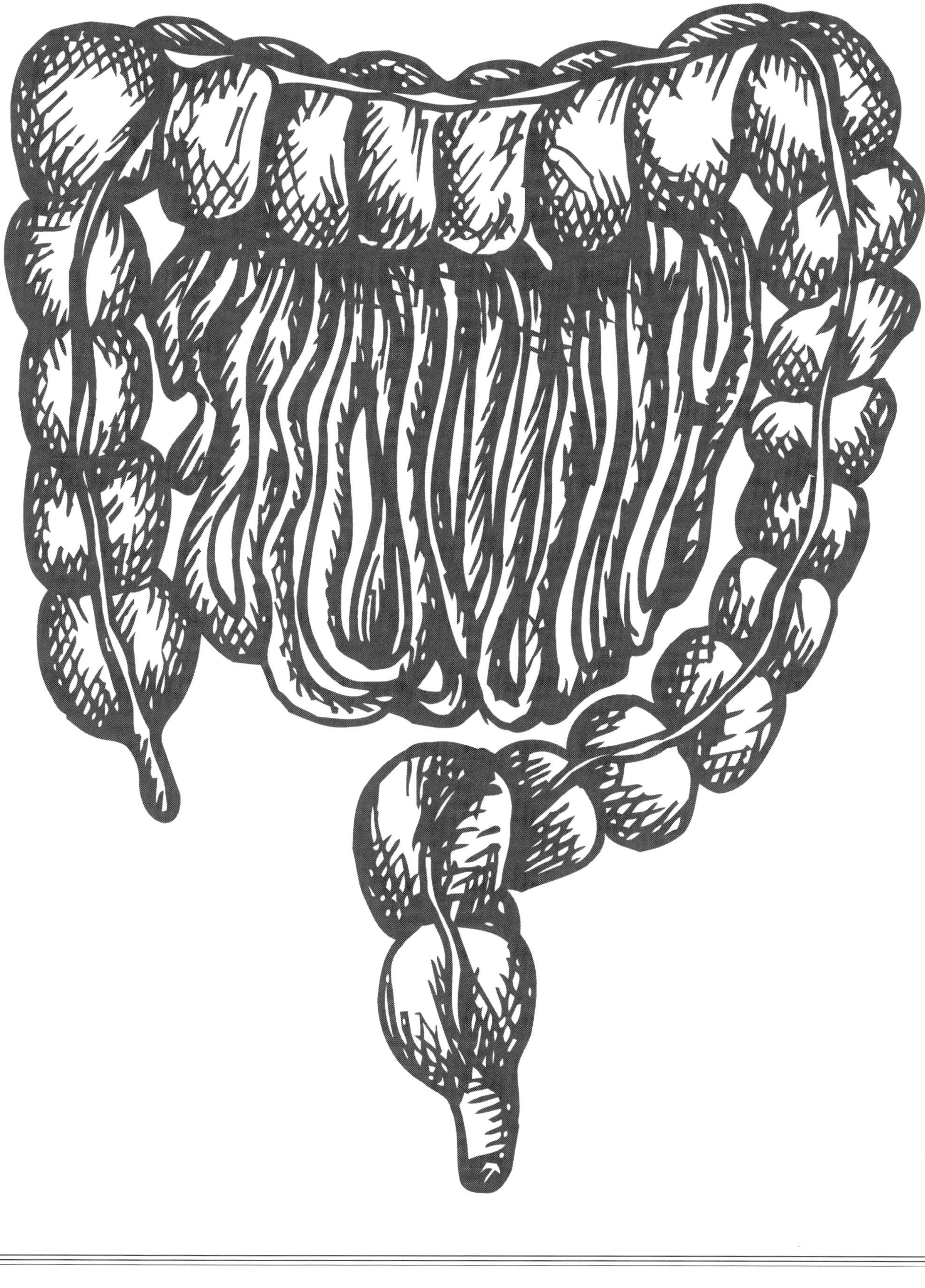

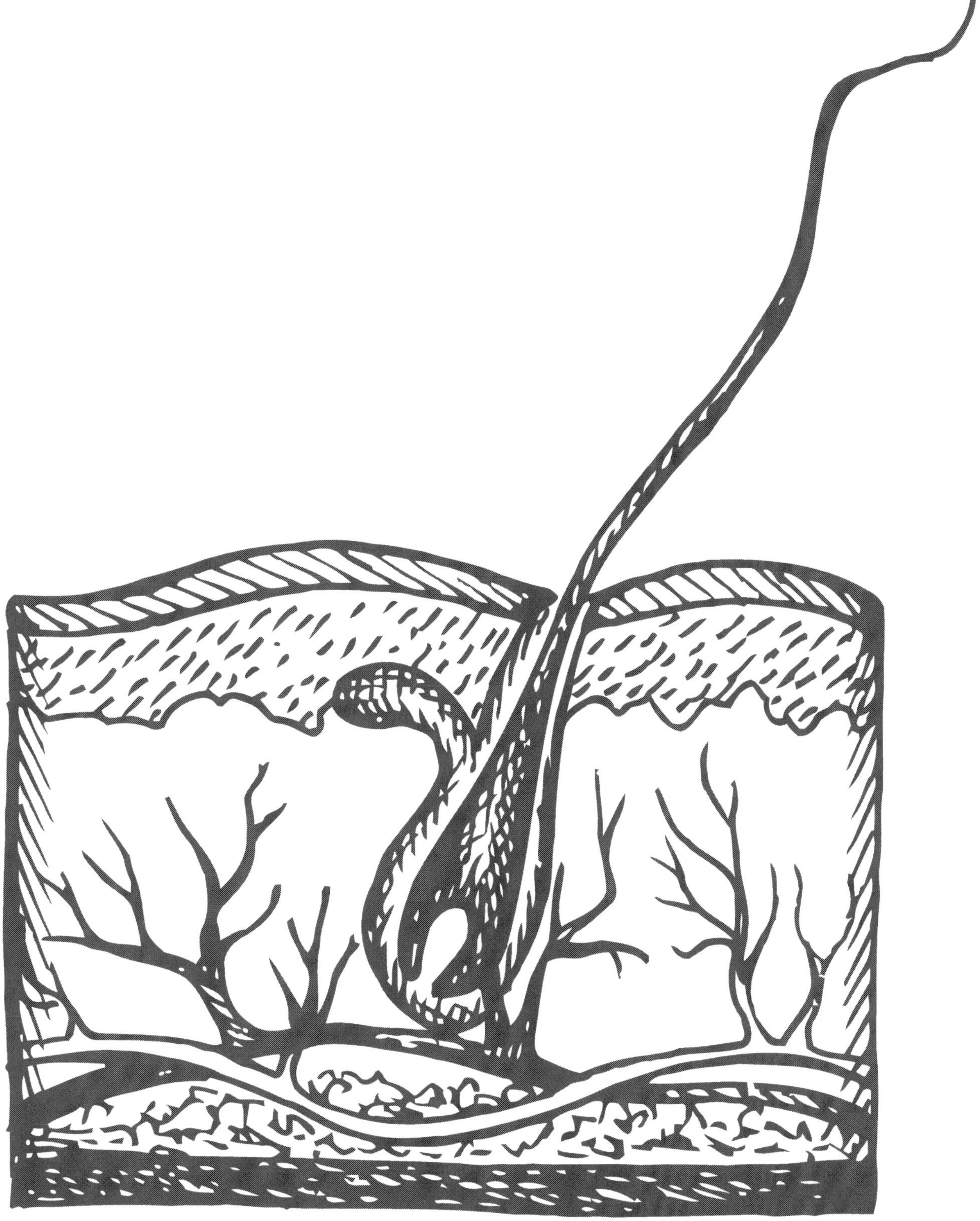

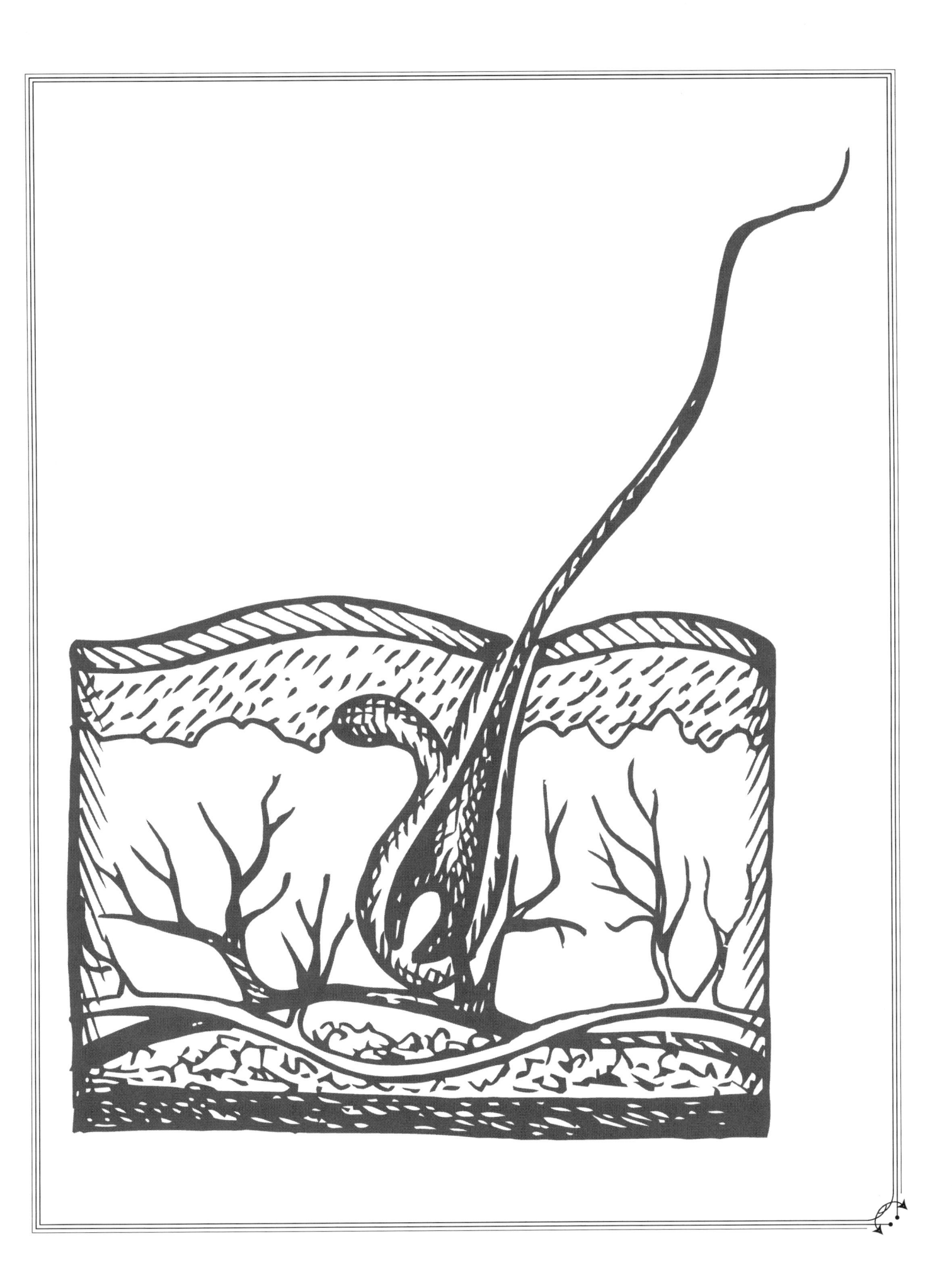

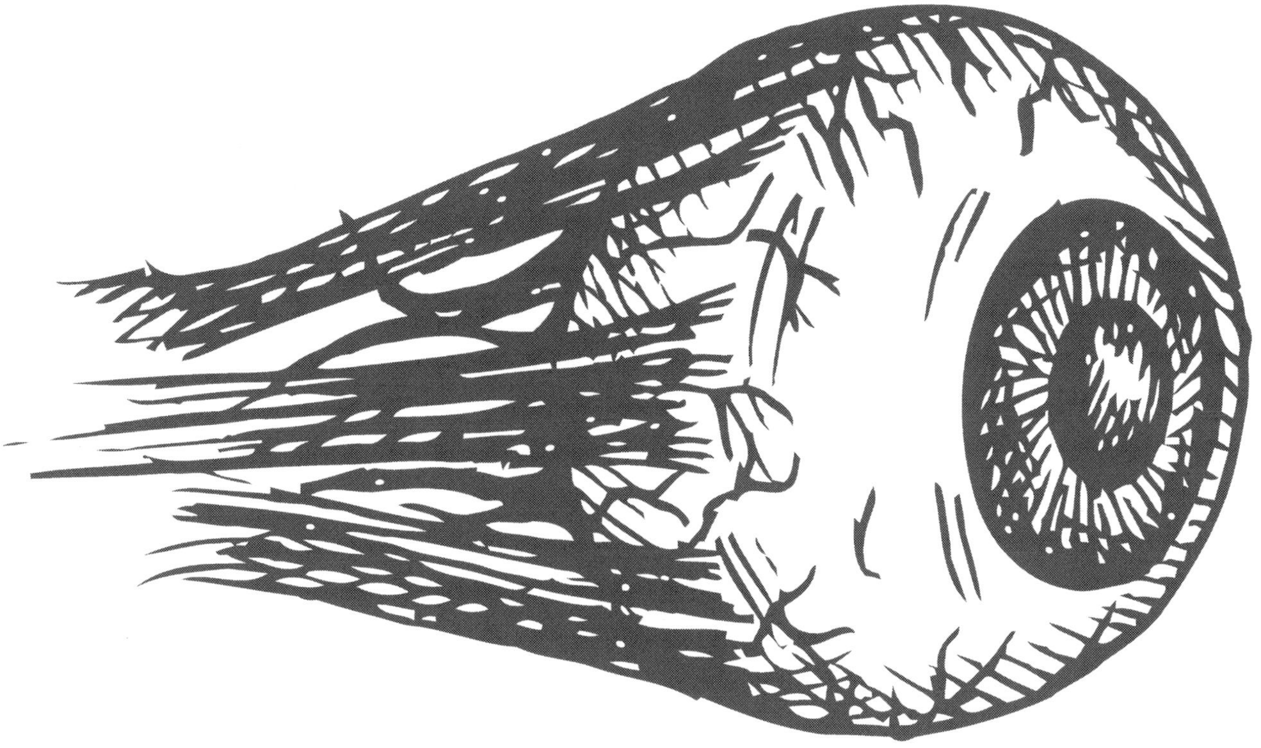

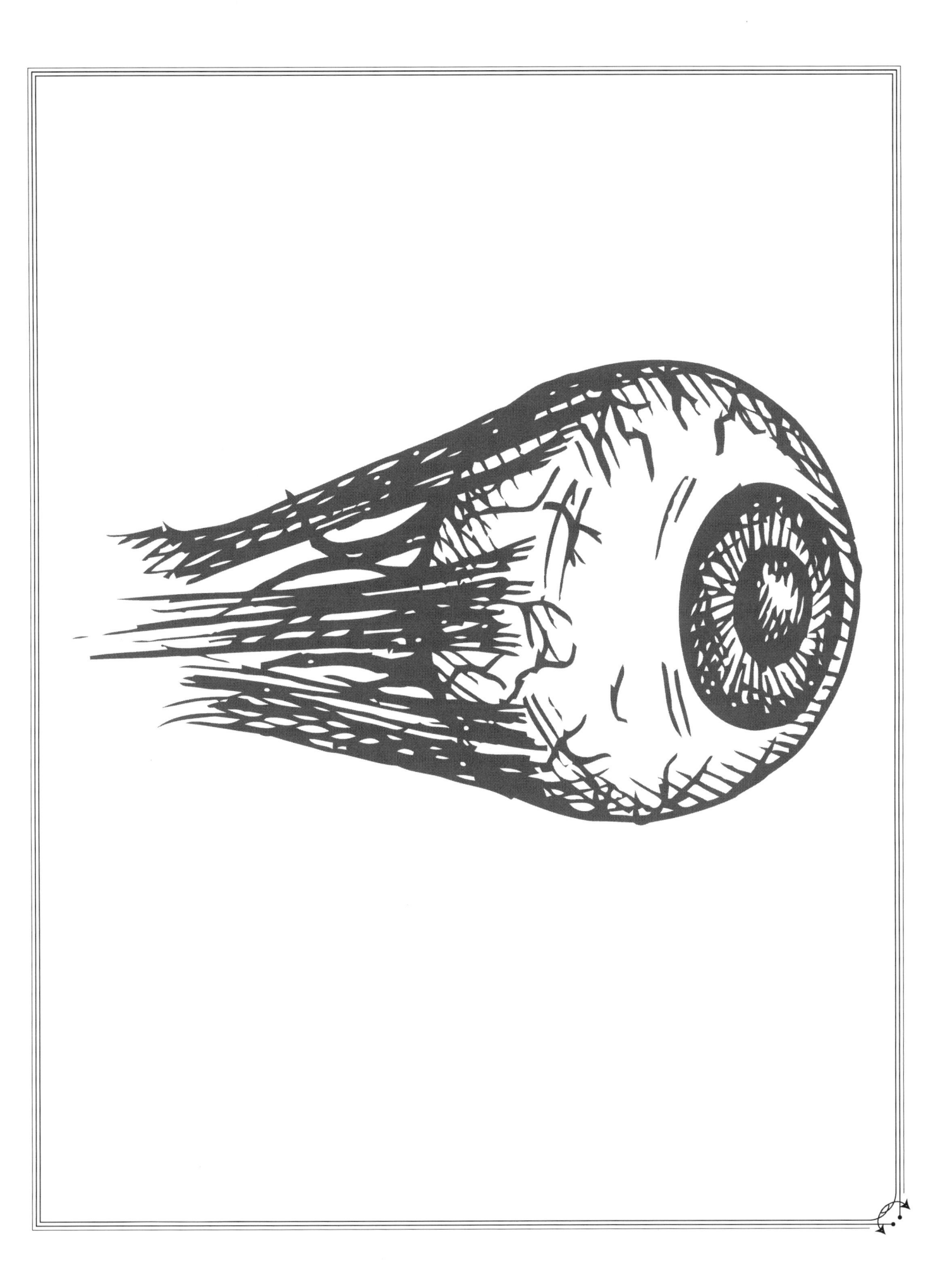

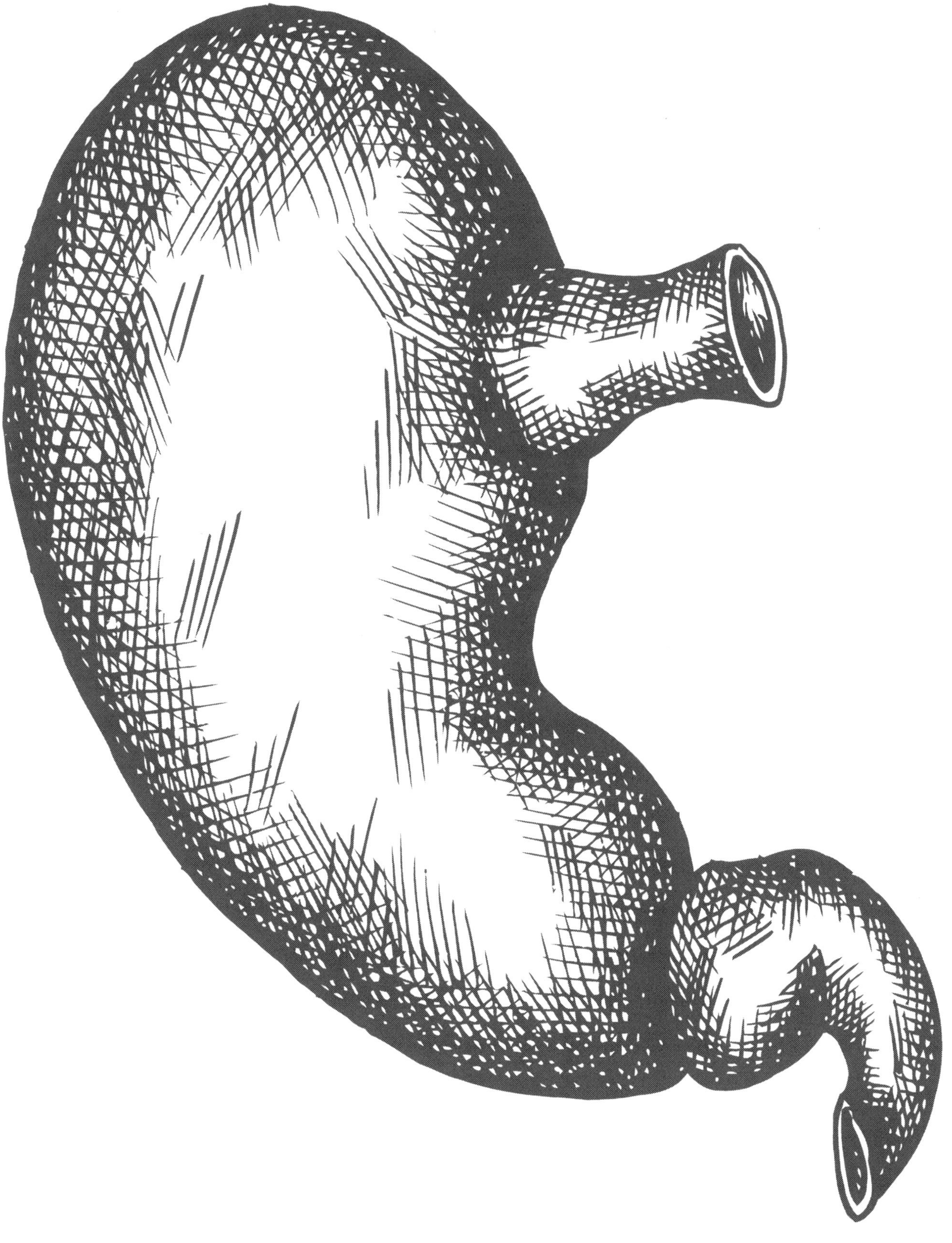

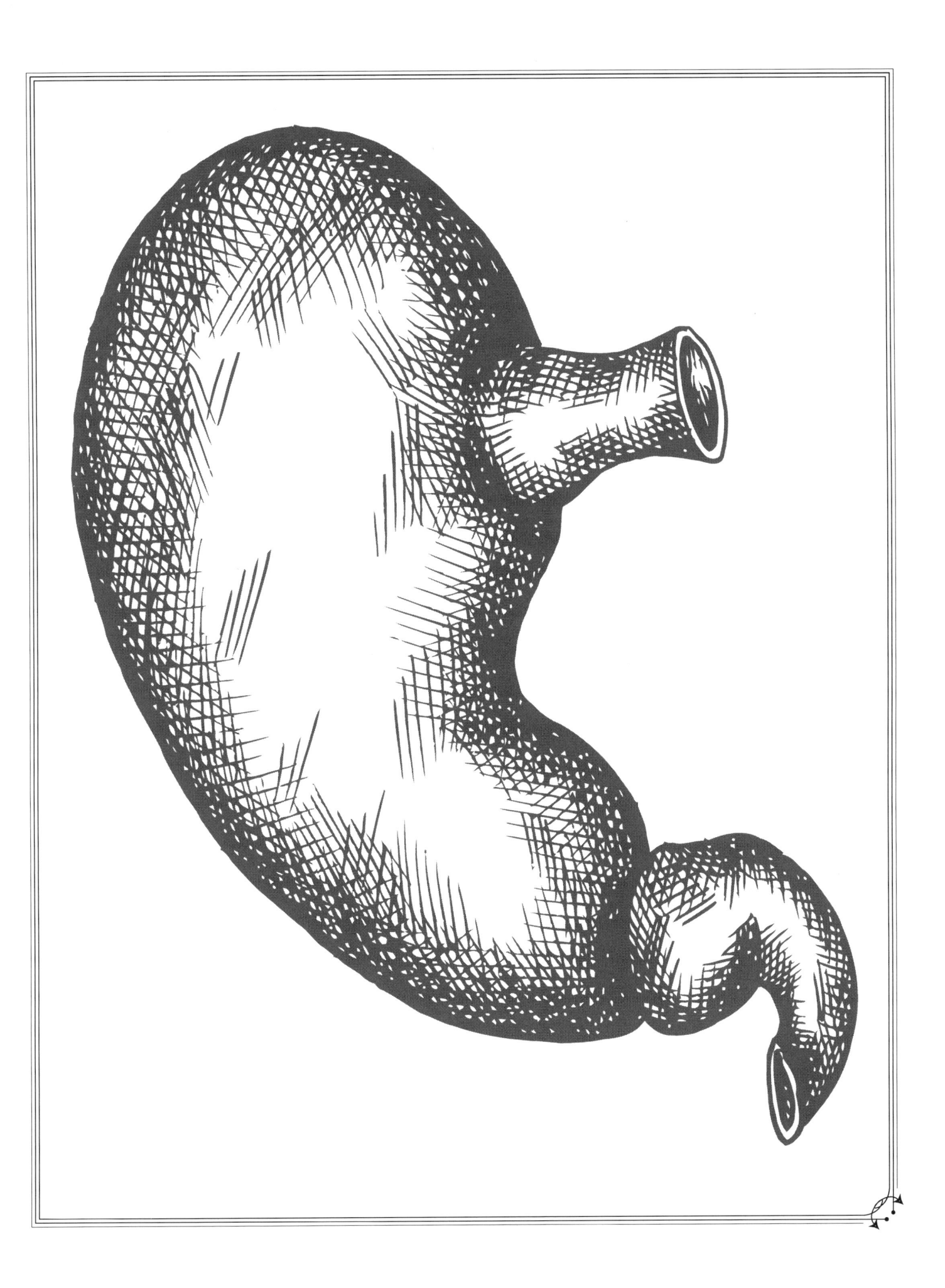

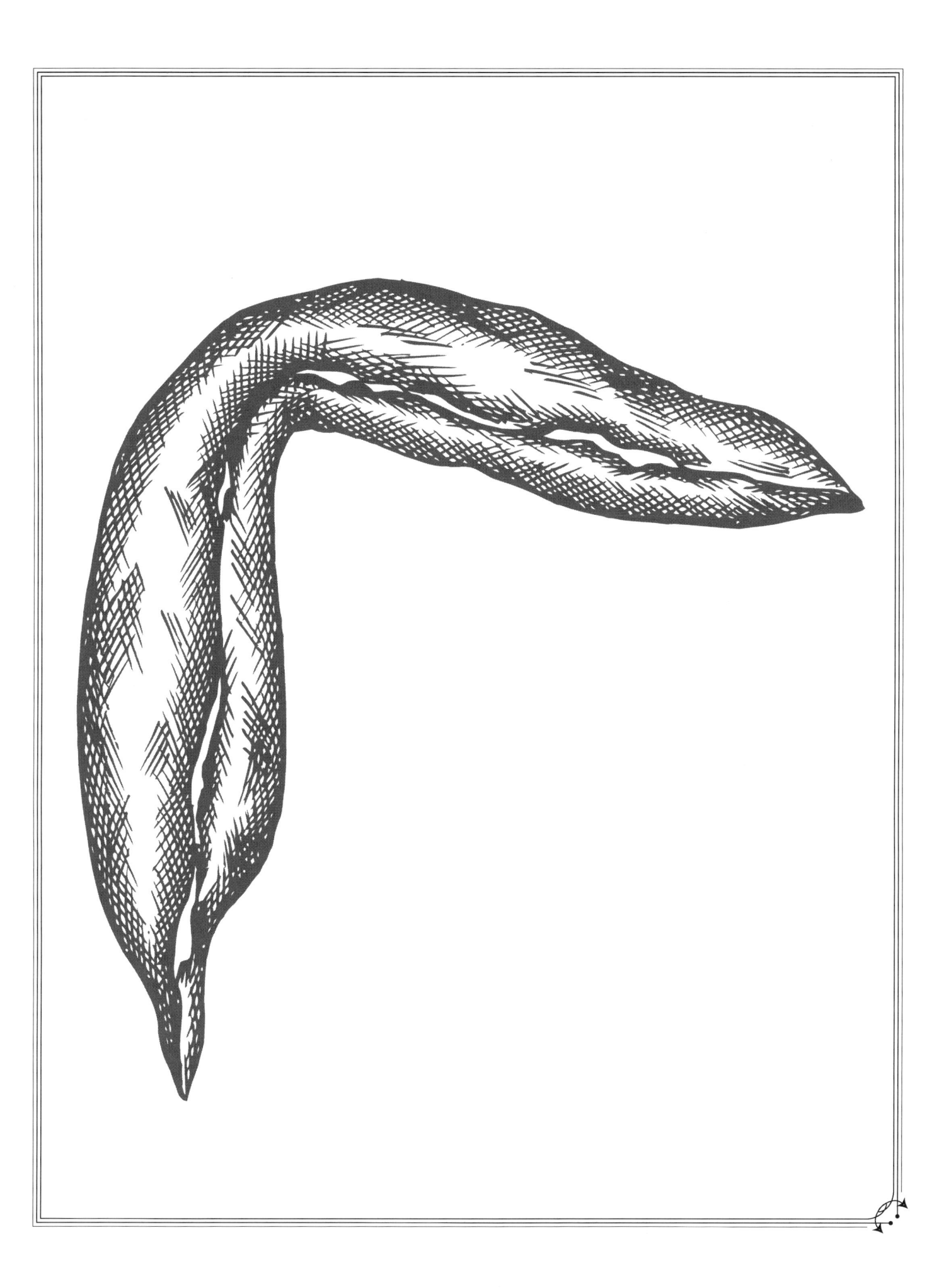

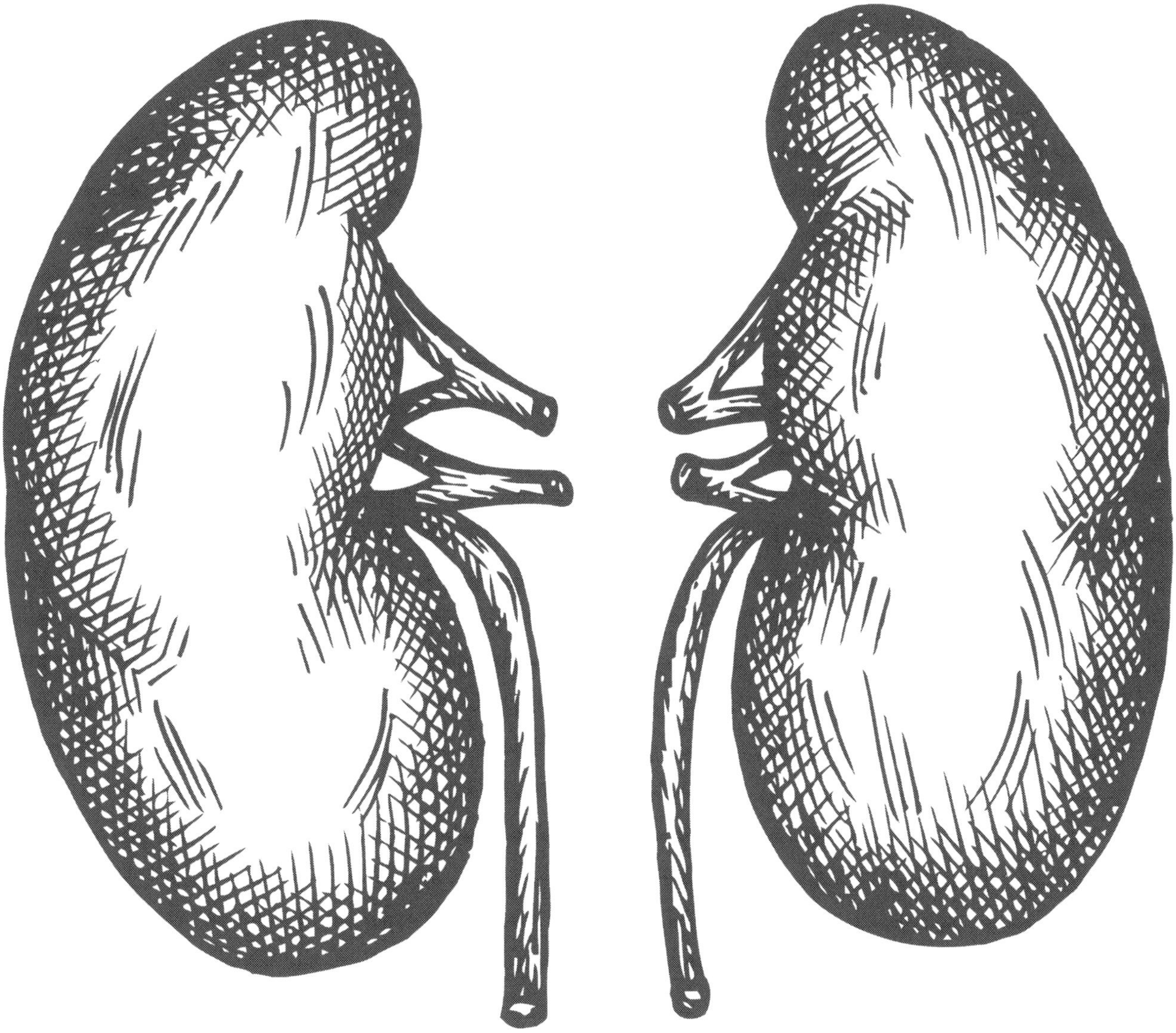

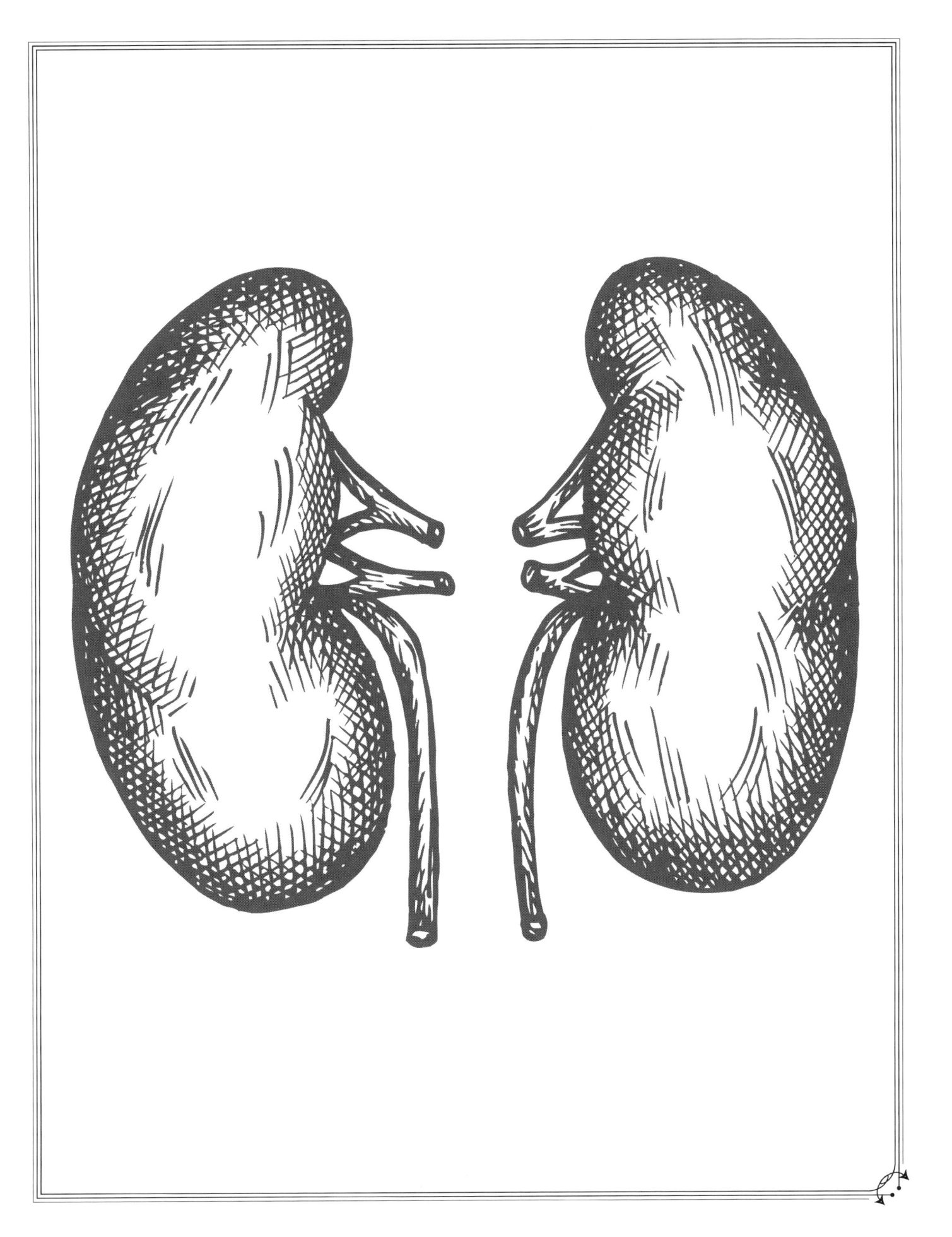

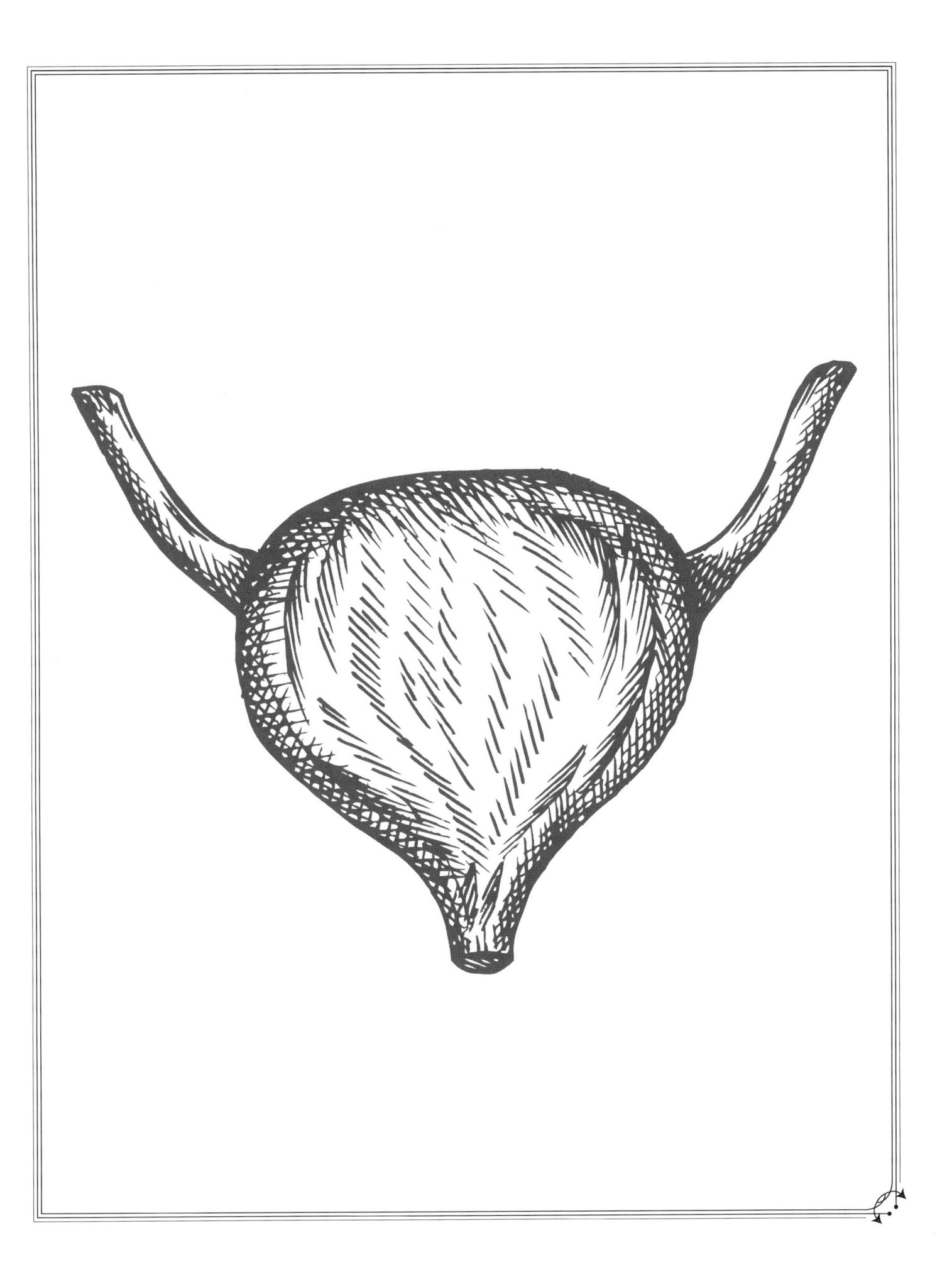

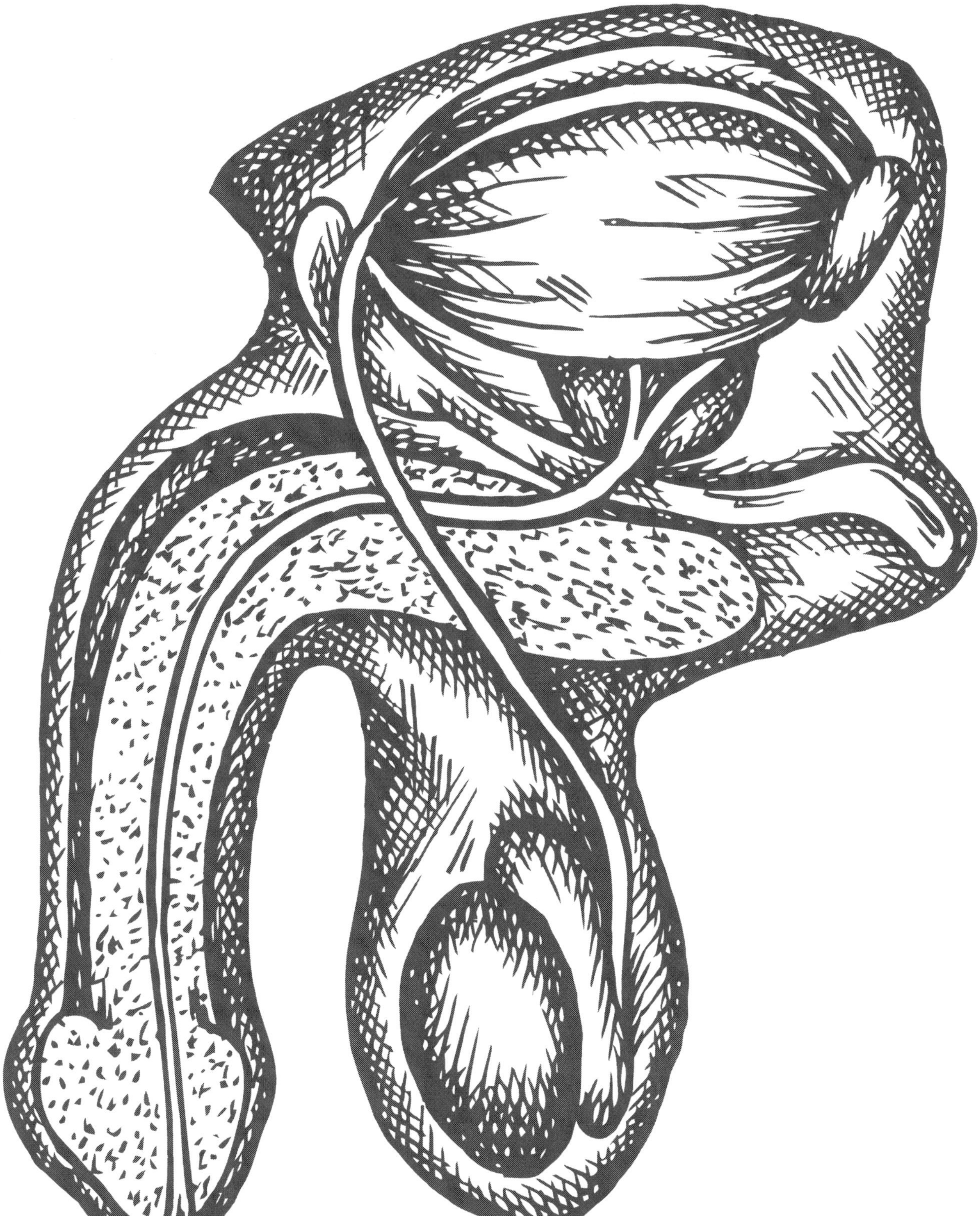

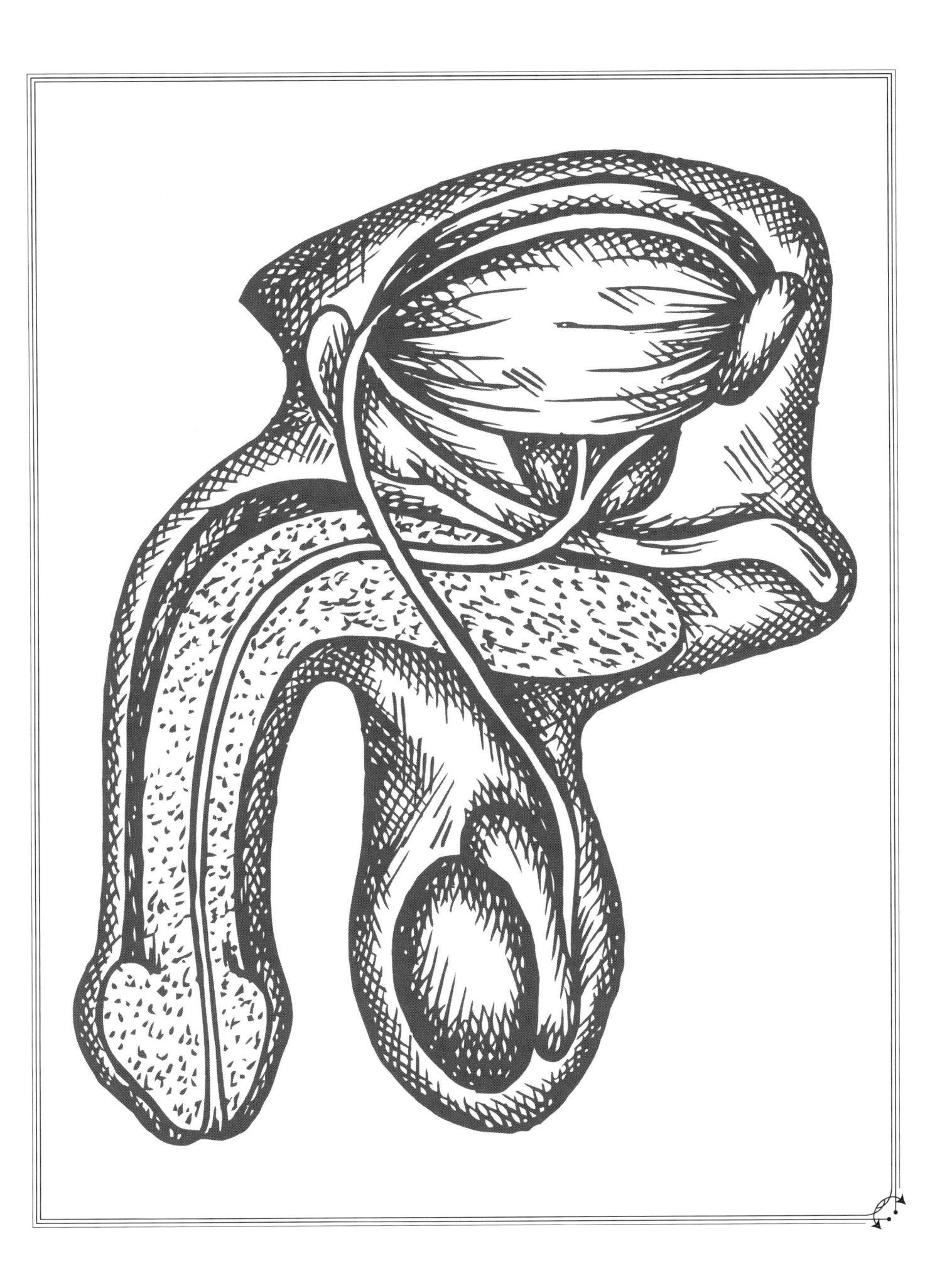

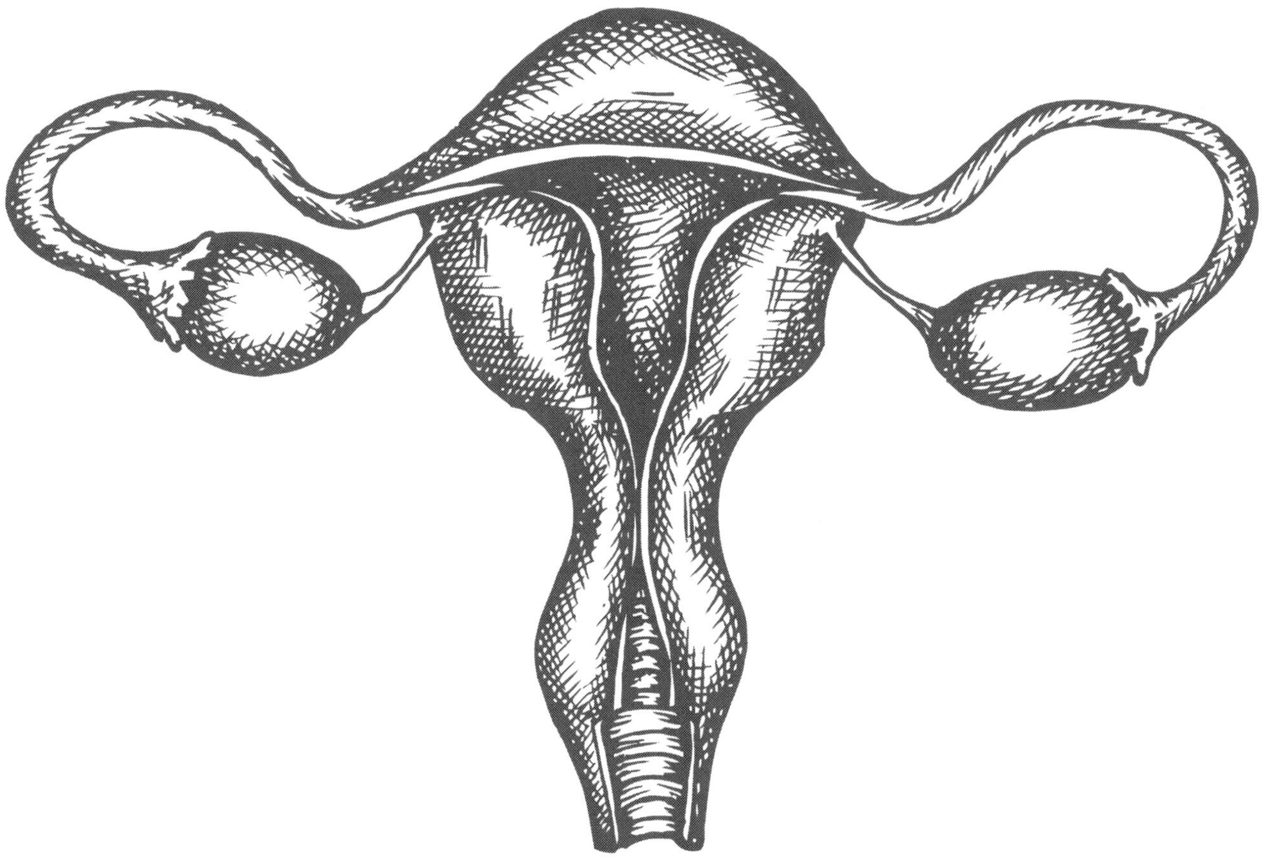

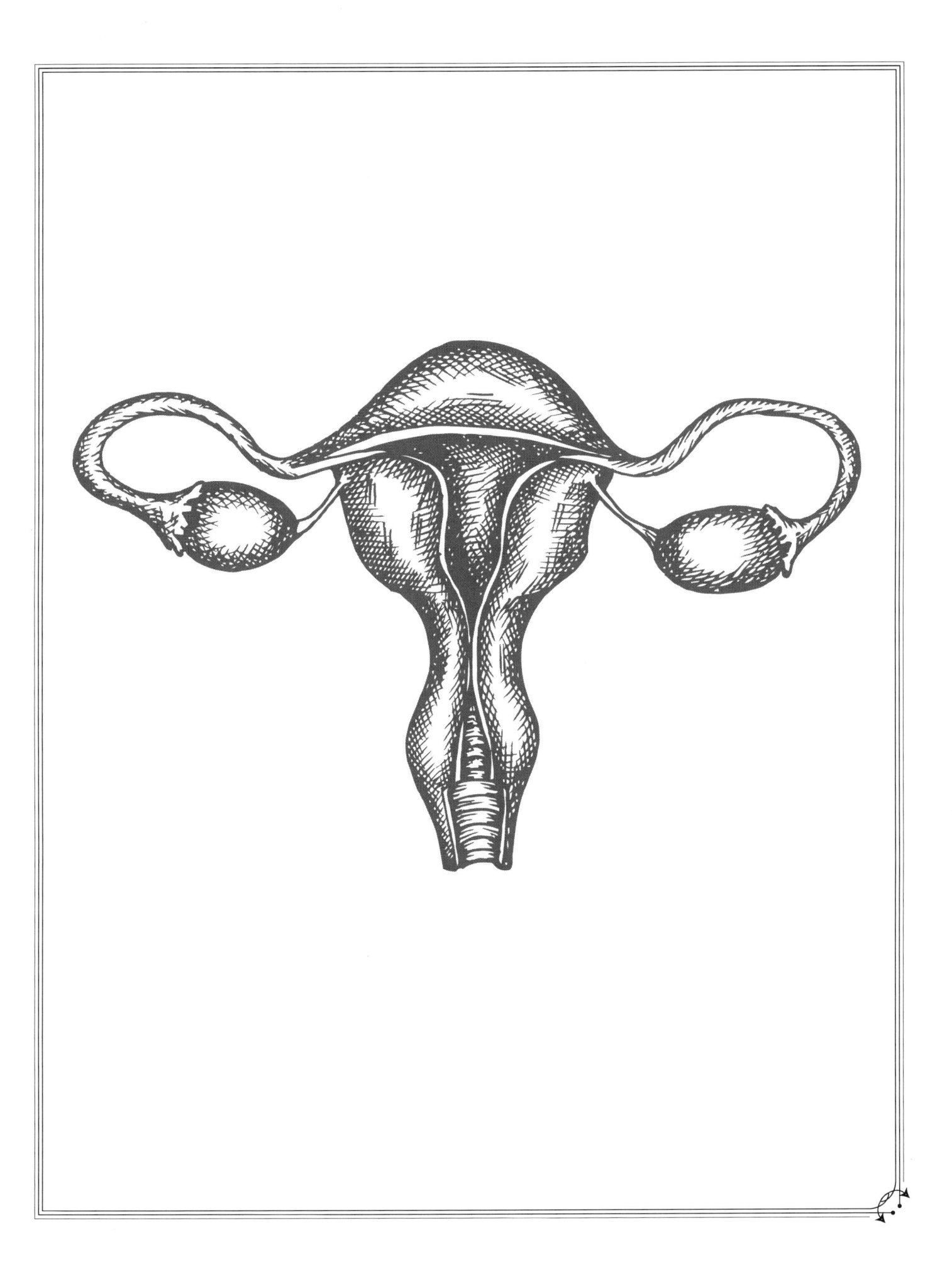

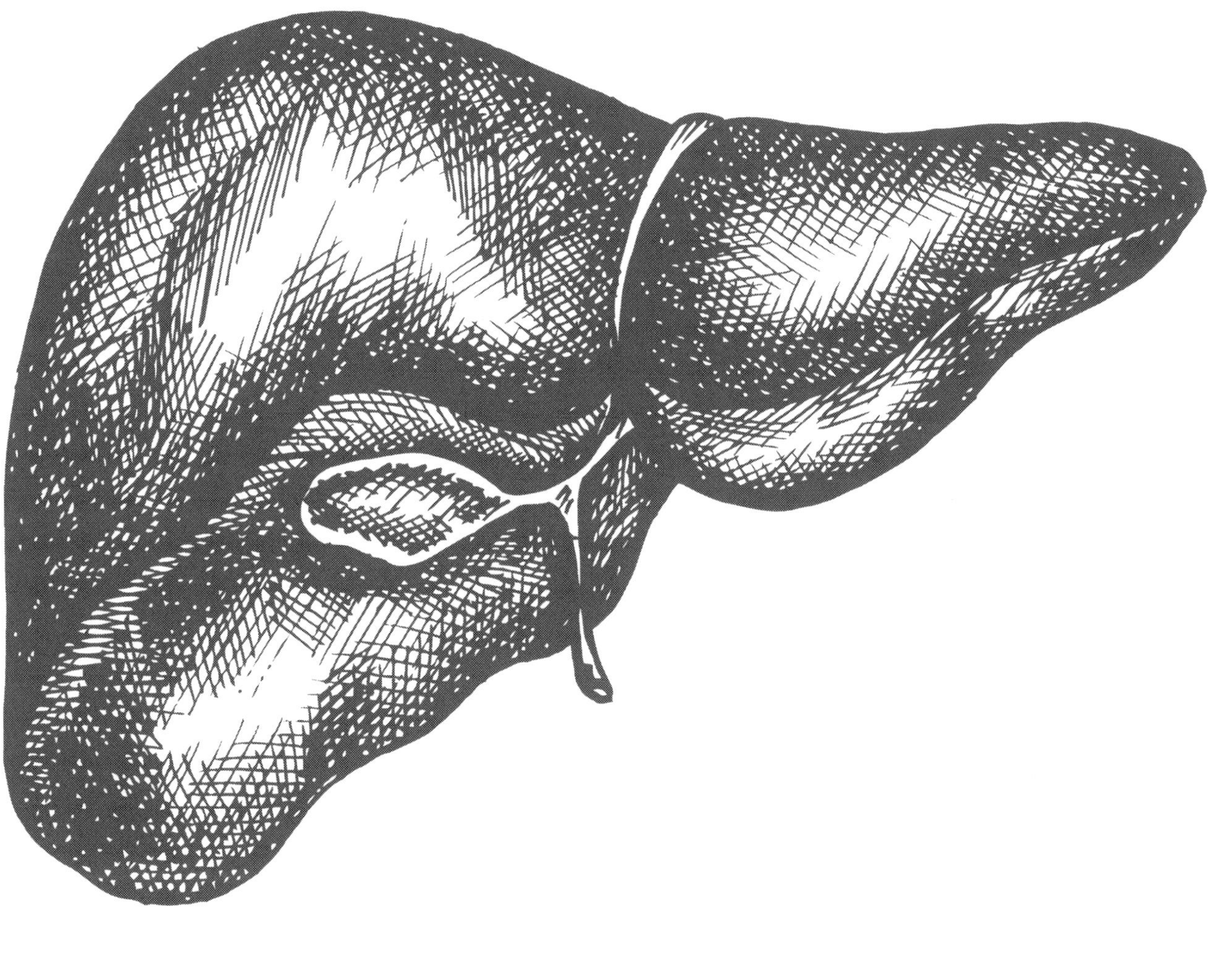

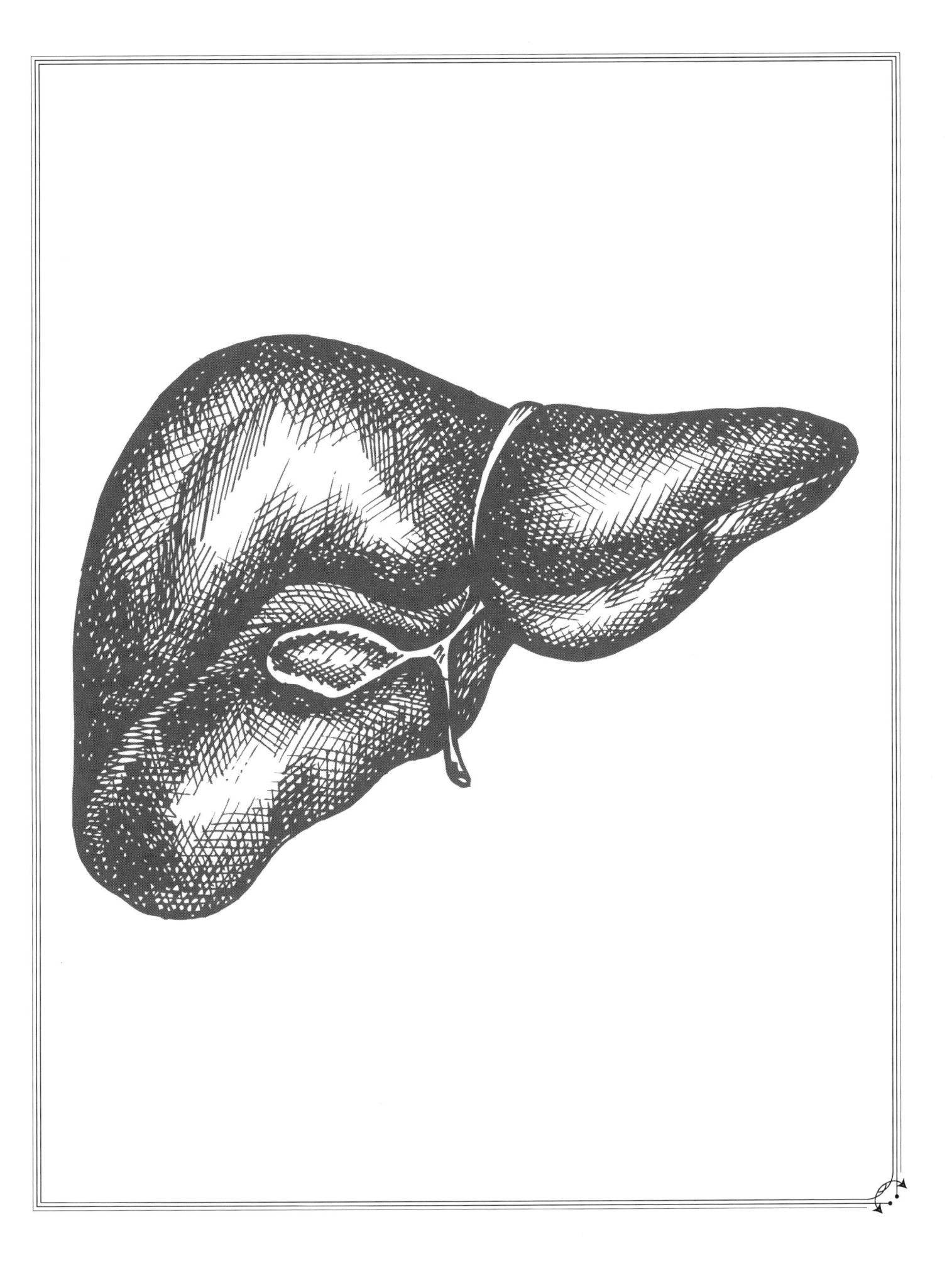

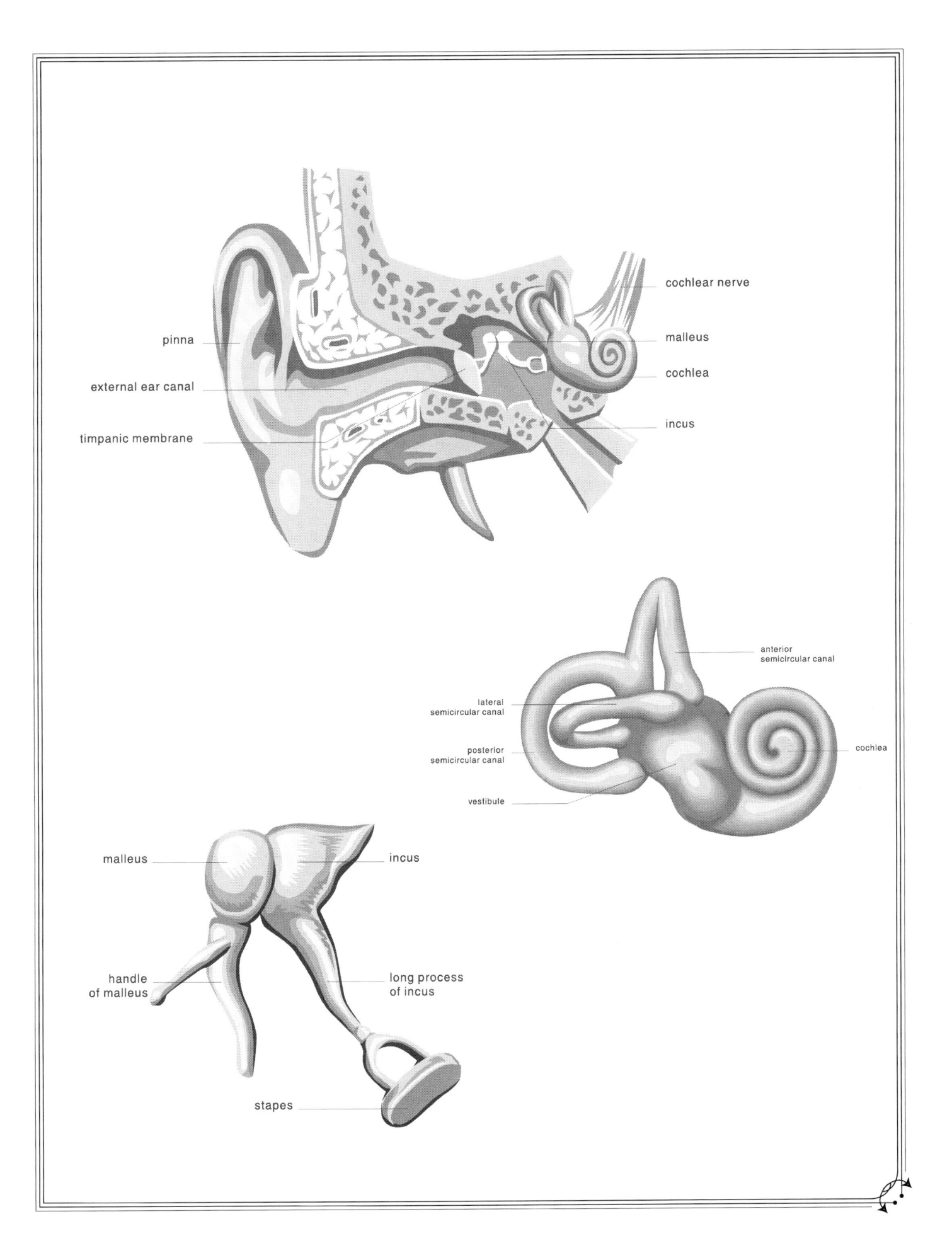

- pinna
- external ear canal
- timpanic membrane
- cochlear nerve
- malleus
- cochlea
- incus

- anterior semicircular canal
- lateral semicircular canal
- posterior semicircular canal
- vestibule
- cochlea

- malleus
- incus
- handle of malleus
- long process of incus
- stapes

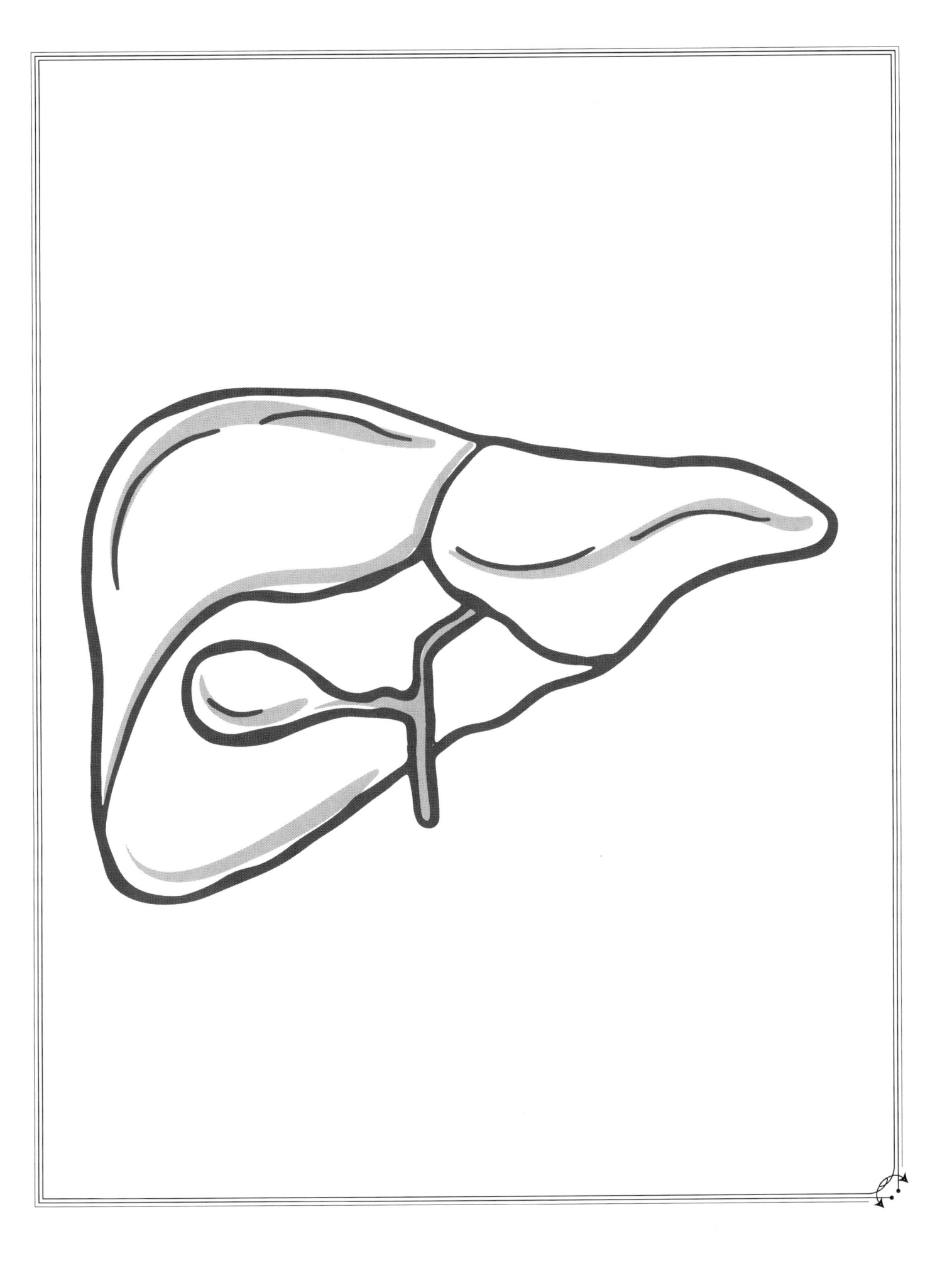

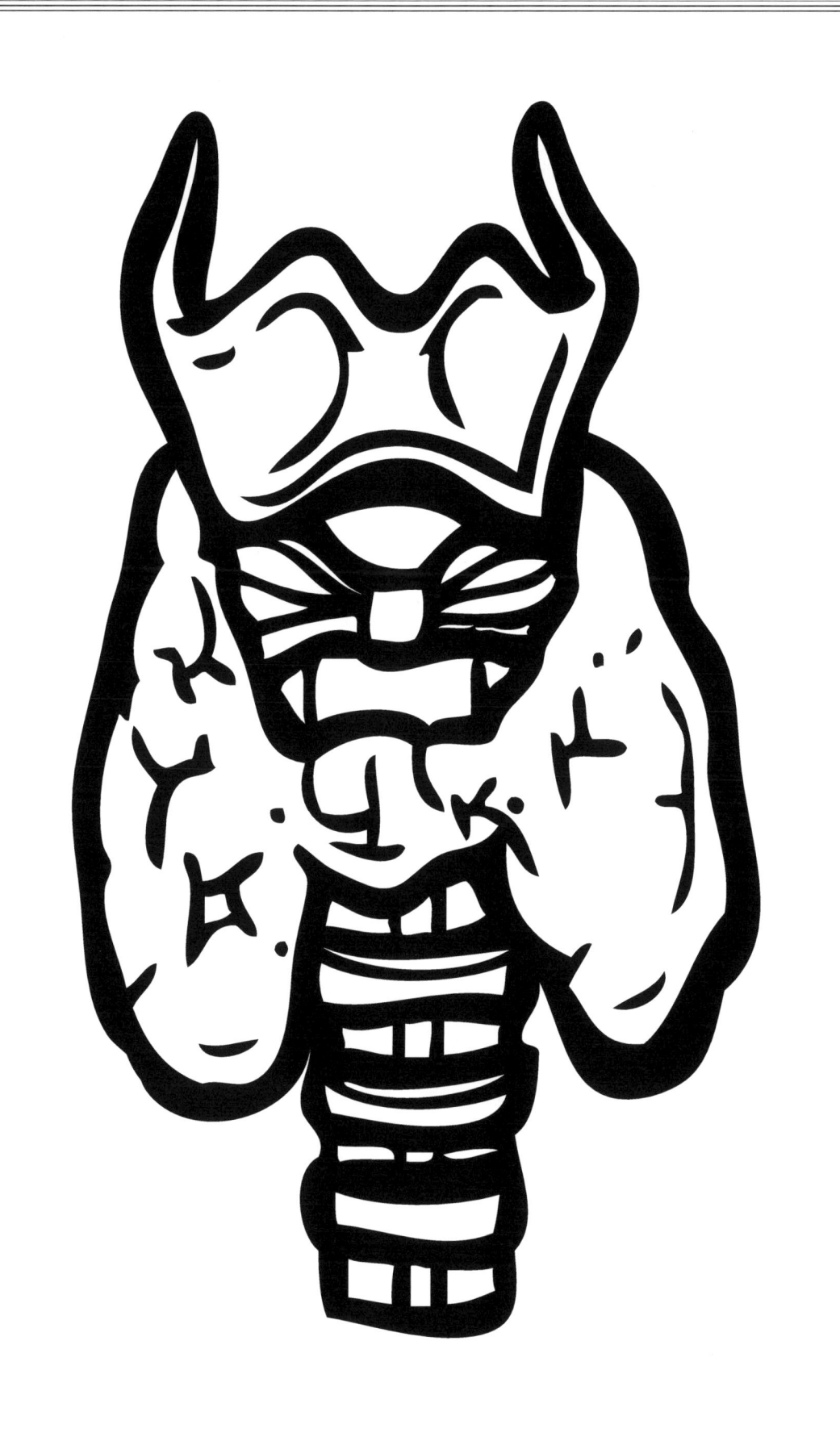

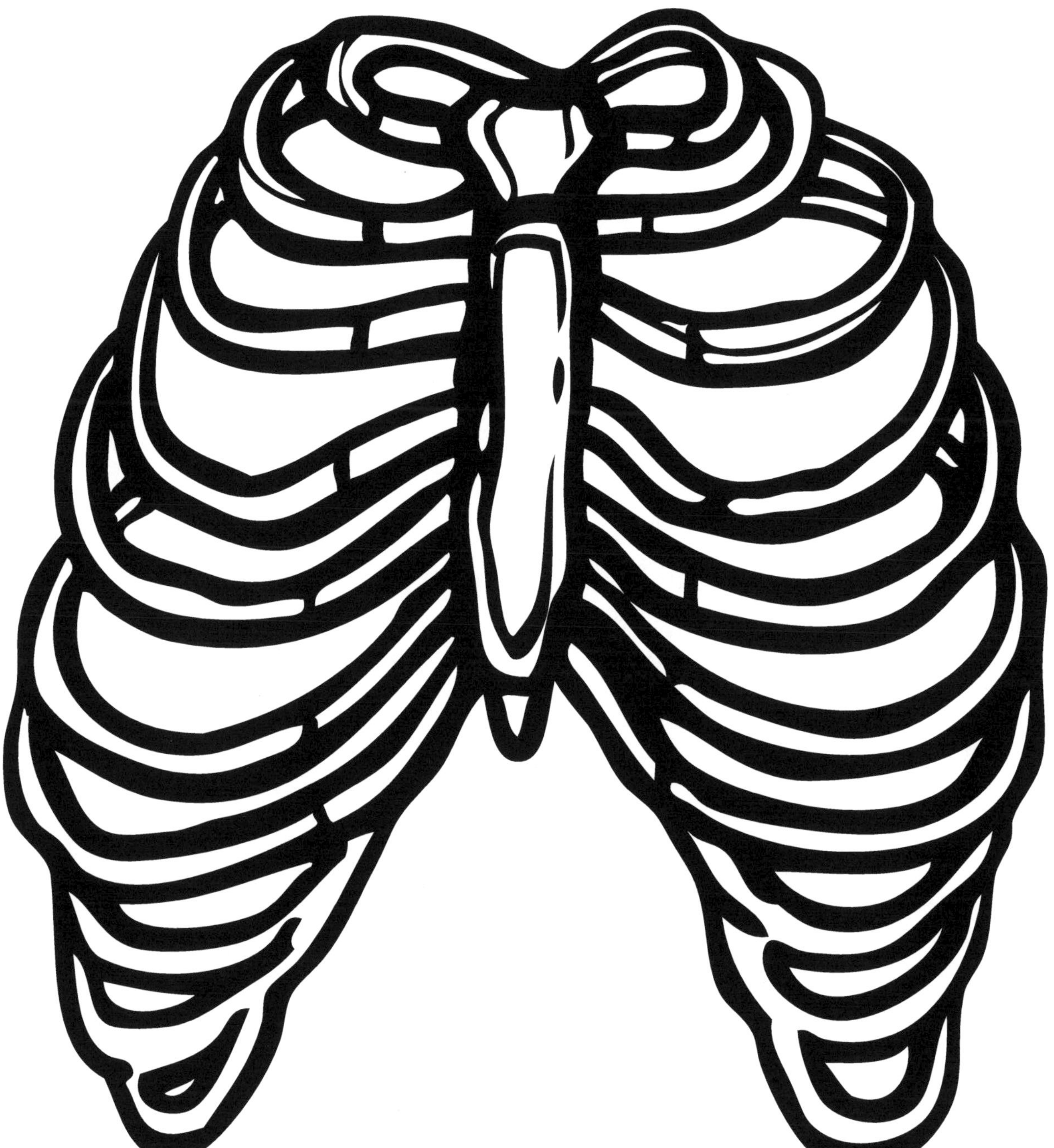

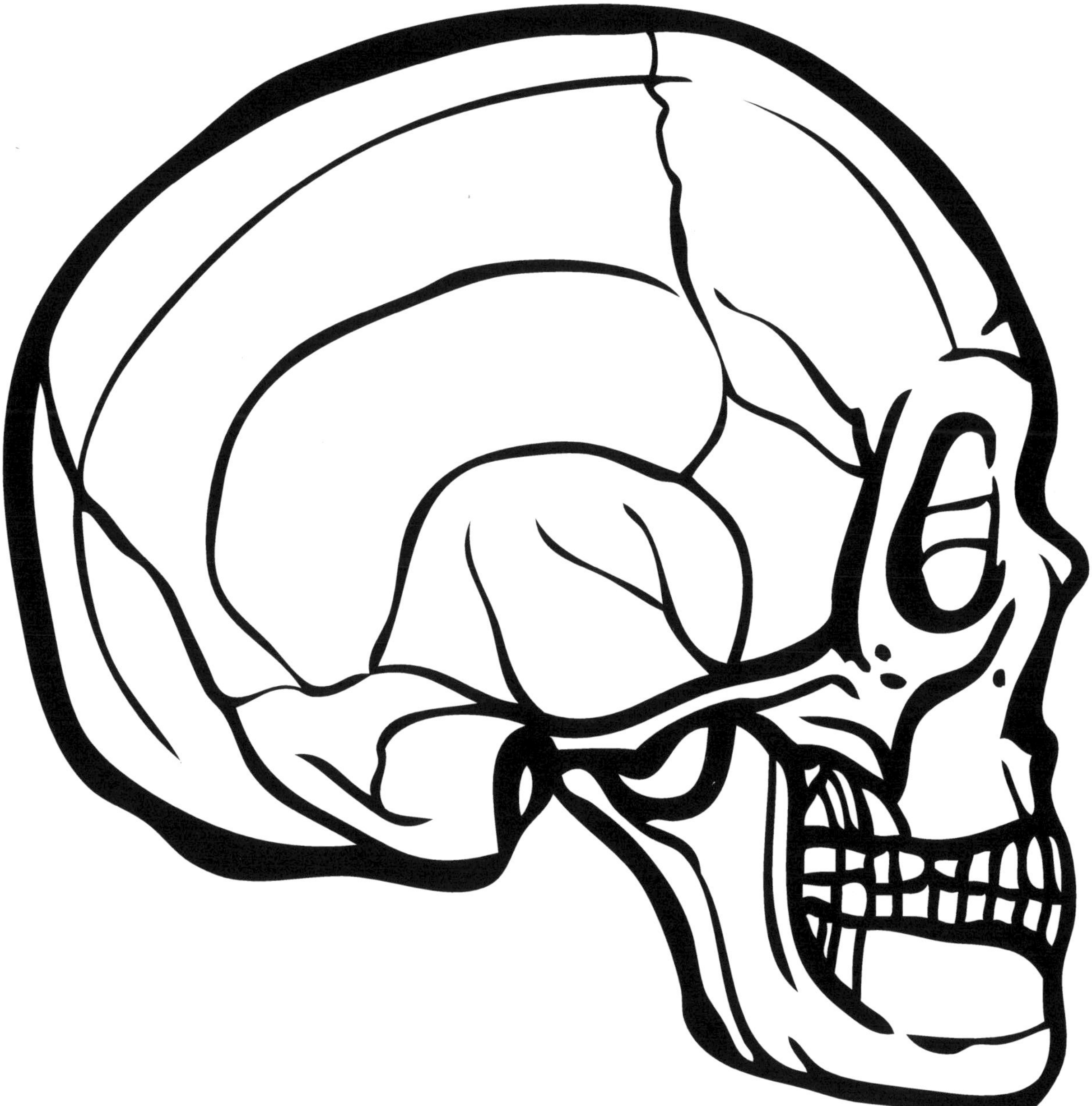

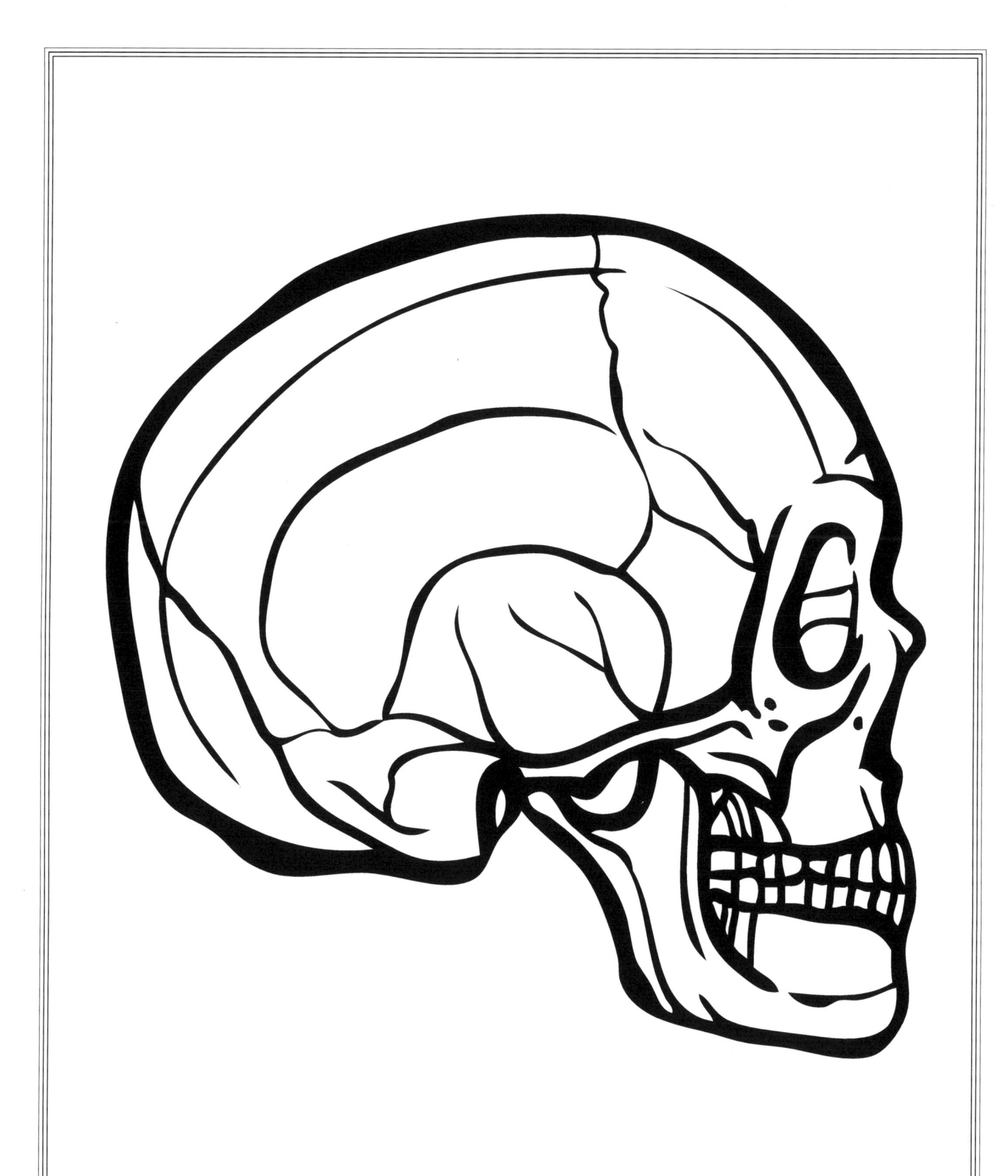

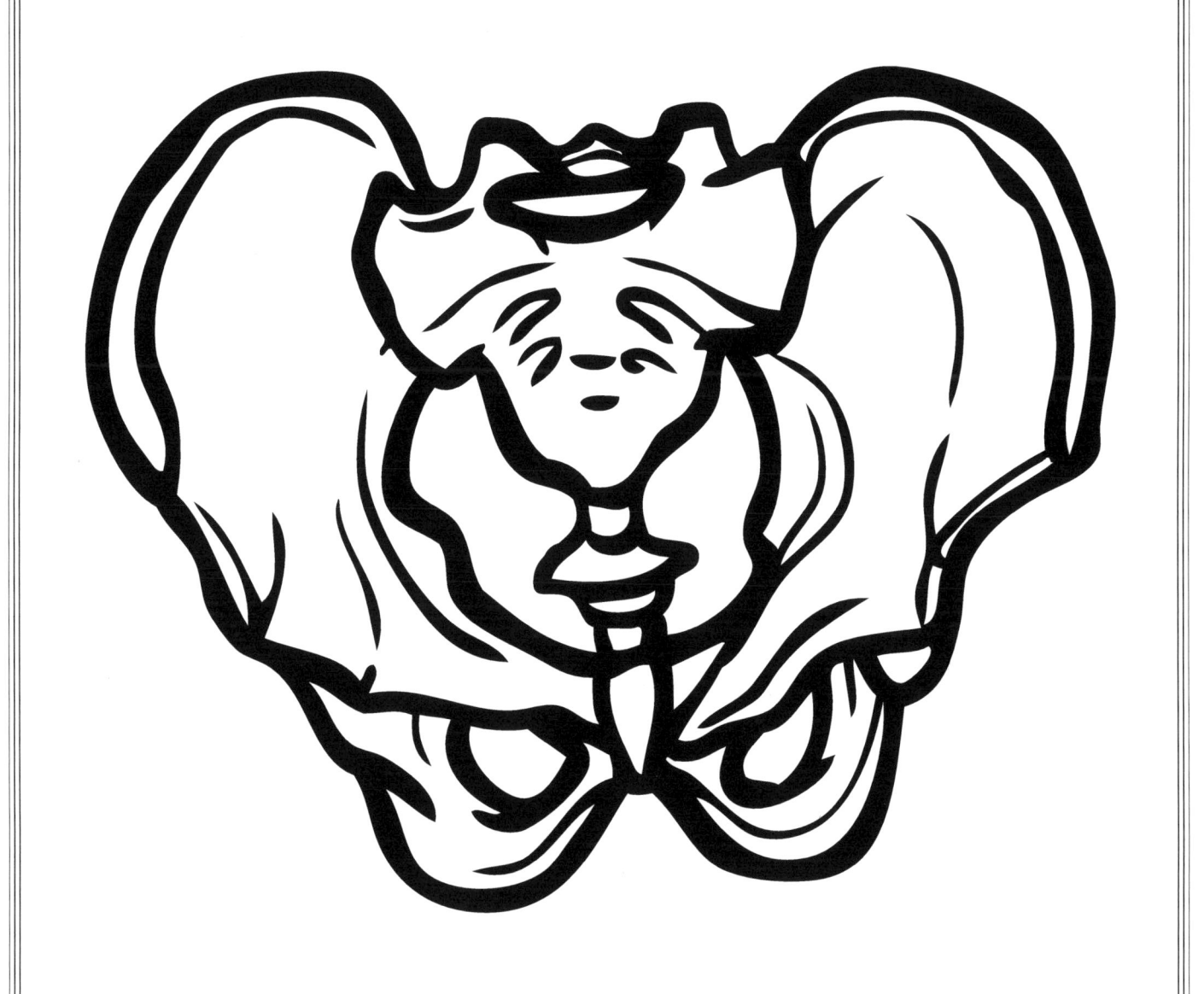

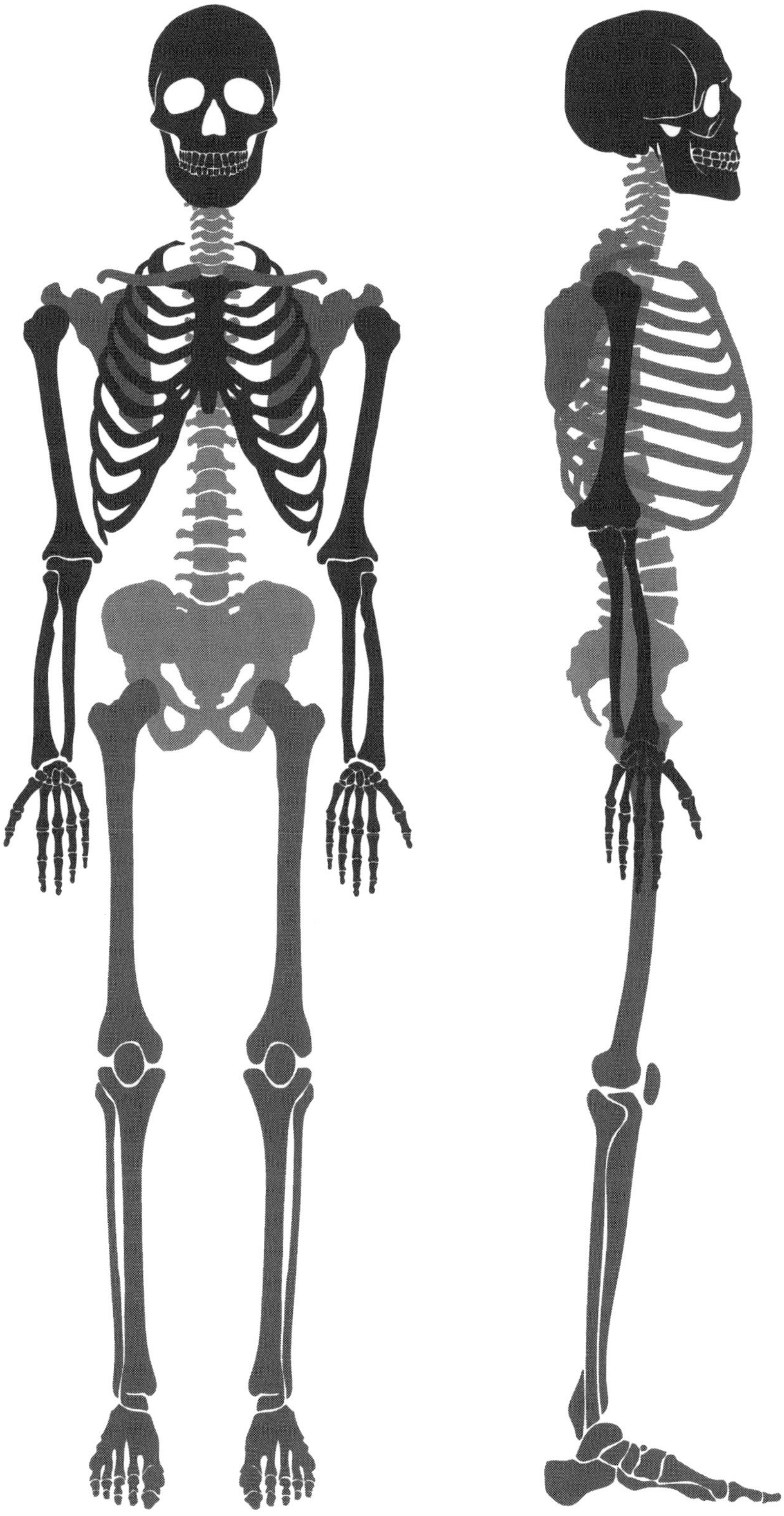

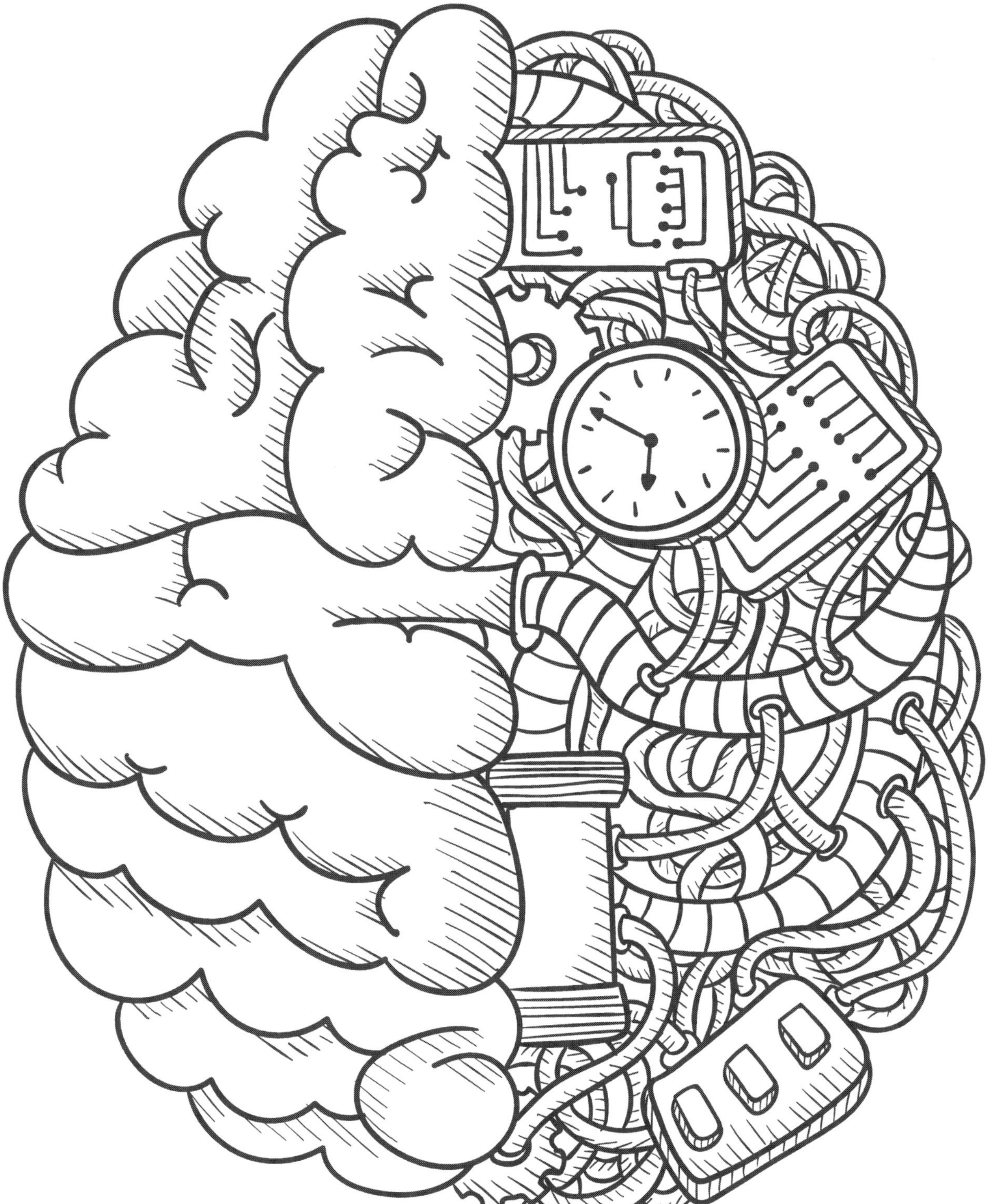

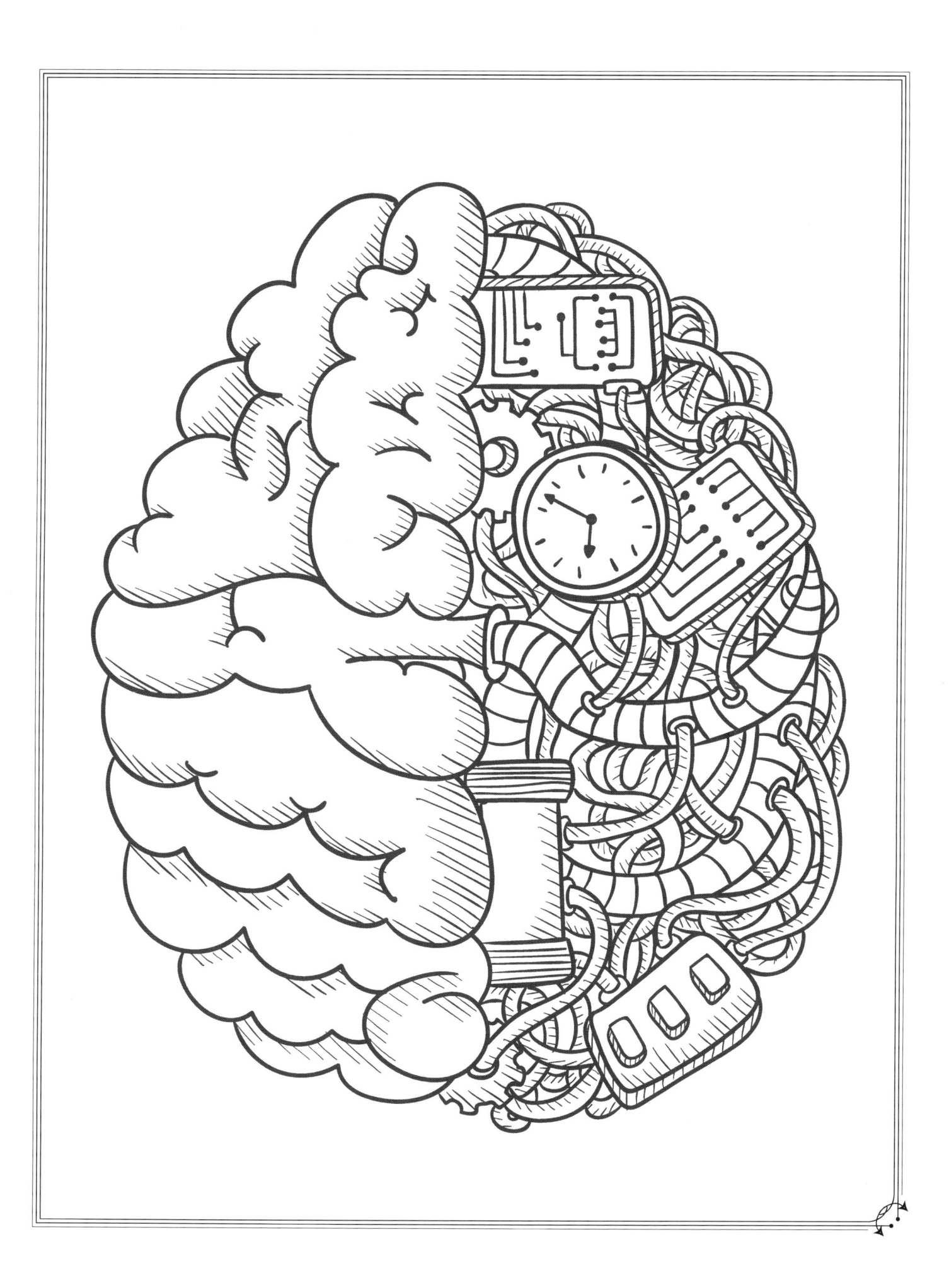

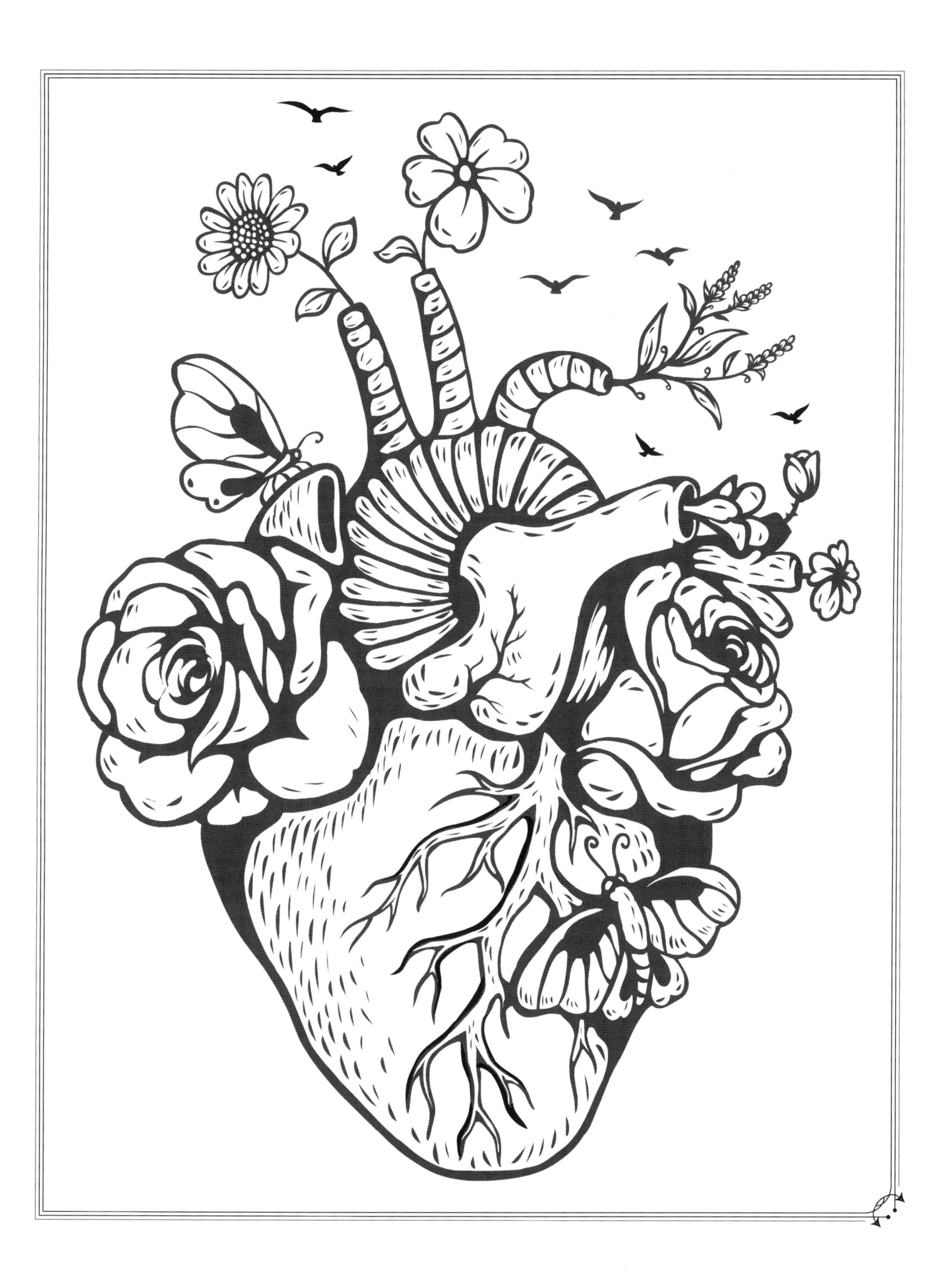

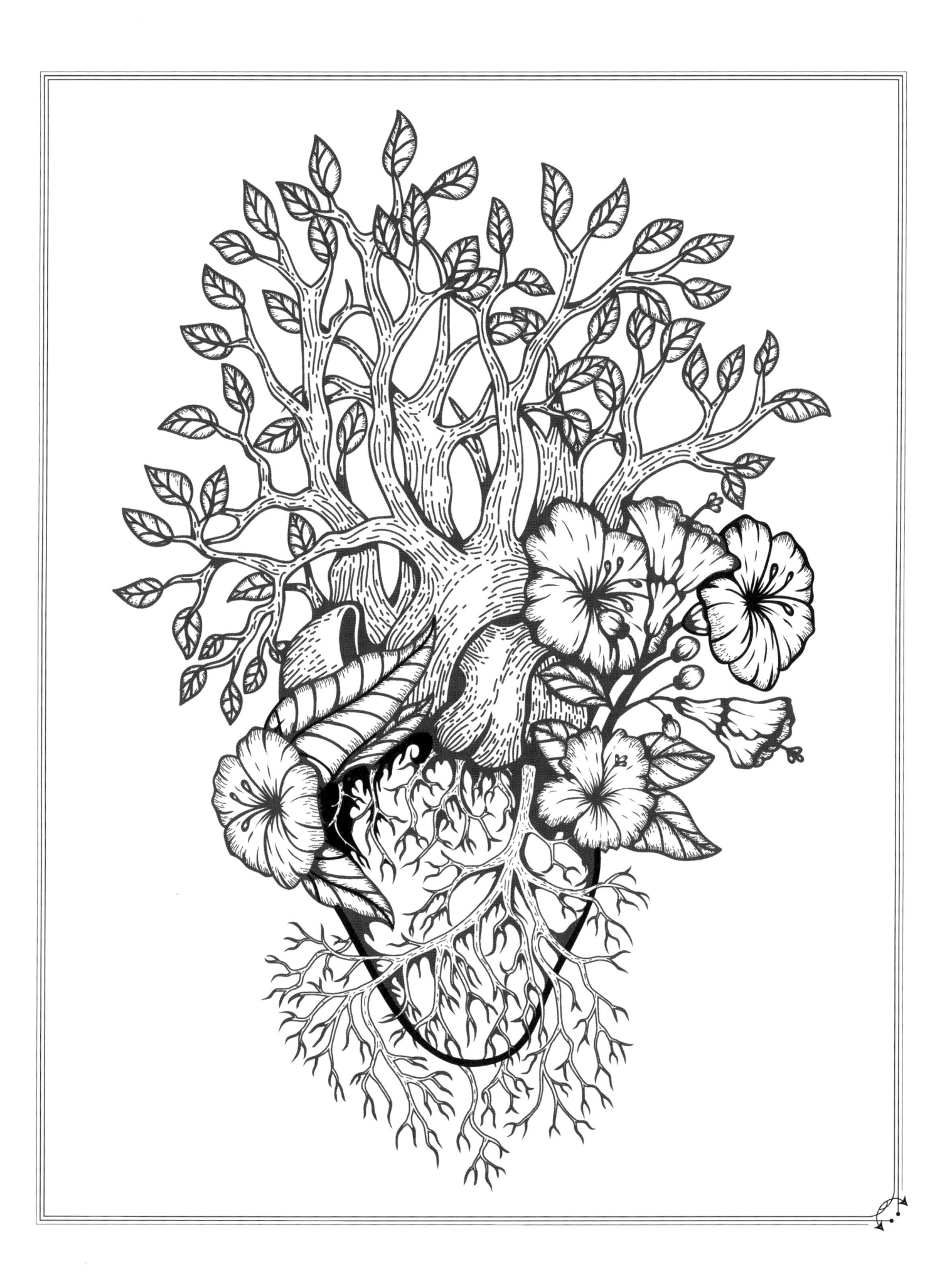

Made in United States
Orlando, FL
14 May 2022